Faces of Promise

Looking Beyond Autism

Faces of Promise

Looking Beyond Autism

Richard Ehrlich   Barbara Firestone

Dignity,
hope,
opportunity,
and love
are the birthrights
of all children.

We dedicate *Faces of Promise* to the children
and their families. Let us do all that we can to
help ensure that all young people living with
autism can experience their birthrights.

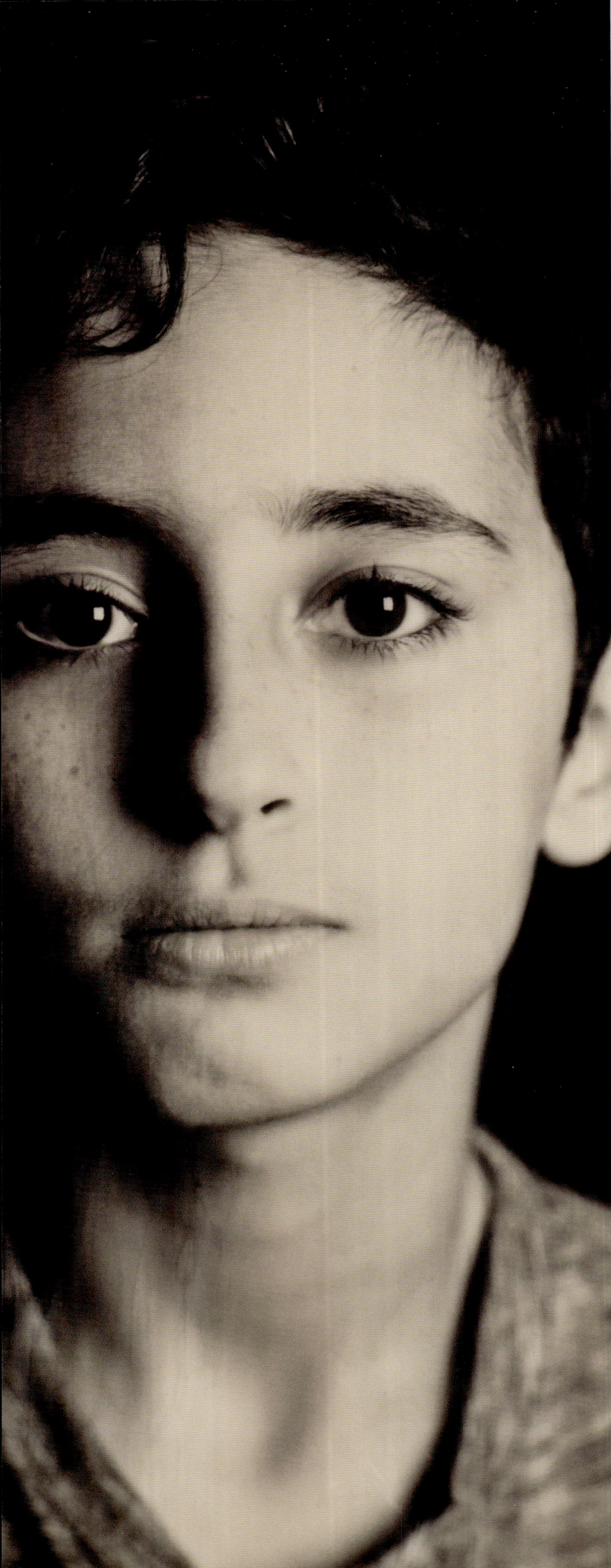

Preface

The genesis of this project emanated from the suggestion by a mother of a child with an autism spectrum disorder. She was perusing images from my recent *Face The Music* project[1] — photographs of recognizable musicians depicting intense emotional states. Sharing with me the challenges she and her family face having a child with autism, she entreated me to consider a project that would illustrate the dignity of these children and their captivating qualities, and serve to counteract the uninformed and erroneous stereotypes many hold about autism. Her passion and sincerity galvanized me to pursue this challenge. I was joined in the *Faces of Promise* effort by Barbara Firestone, who is highly regarded for her longstanding commitment to children with autism and their families. I am most grateful to Barbara for her sensitivity and understanding that added such an important dimension to this endeavor.

Despite the more than four decades of working as a physician, surgeon and educator, nothing prepared me for what I was to experience meeting these children.

The use of the 20"x24" Polaroid Camera — of which remain only 3 in use worldwide — with its mysterious aura and almost surreal depth of field, added special and ethereal nuances to the portraits. This historic, soon-to-be-extinct camera afforded unique and fascinating images, capturing, in portraiture, the essence and beauty of these children. The juxtaposition of the 20"x24" Polaroid images with similarly captivating Canon digital images and several 8"x10" black and white Polaroids evokes a countervailing feeling tone and context.

What I experienced and came to appreciate was a profound understanding of what these dedicated parents have come to know — that although their children have autism, they are not defined by it — they are much more than a label. I saw in detail the uniqueness of each one of these children and came to recognize that individuality is one of their defining qualities.

As I peeled the first Polaroid image from the back of the camera, the child's mother cried and told me the photo had brought light into her world again. It was a moment I will never forget.

It has been a transcendent, even transformative experience, and I feel privileged to have been granted access to the private world of these children and their families.

As both a physician and a photographer, I rarely get an opportunity to be so extraordinarily affected by either patients or photographic subjects.

Faces of Promise has been a life-altering experience for which I am profoundly grateful. It has also instilled in me an overwhelming respect for *The Help Group*, *The Bay School,* and all who serve these children with their uncompromising dedication and tender care.

In reading the statements from parents and children accompanying these portraits, *Faces of Promise* evokes both a very moving and uplifting experience. It resonates as a celebration of all children with autism and their families.

As Cicero proclaimed, "The face is the image of the soul."

And further, "In art, as in life, there are few more pleasurable sights than the human face."[2]

Richard Ehrlich, M.D.

1 Richard Ehrlich: *Face The Music*. Steidl, 2015.
2 Eric R. Kandel: *The Age of Insight: The Quest to Understand the Unconscious In Art, Mind and Brain: From Vienna 1900 to the Present*. Random House 2012.

Preface

About two-and-a-half years ago, Rick Ehrlich approached me with an idea he had to contribute to the acceptance of children with autism through his photography. As an artist, he wanted to capture their beauty and dignity. He asked me if it would be possible for *The Help Group* to participate in an endeavor of this kind. After I gave it some thought, I told him that I would like to proceed with creating a book with him. I have been familiar with his work and have appreciated his sensitivity.

We talked a great deal about autism, how complex it is, and that it is currently estimated to affect 1 in every 68 children in the U.S. I told him that autism is a group of brain-based developmental disorders characterized by impaired social communication and interaction and repetitive behaviors. I explained that the autism spectrum is very broad and that children can have symptoms that range from mild to severe. Each child is unique having varying abilities, challenges, strengths and differences, but all have the potential to make gains when given the educational and therapeutic opportunities tailored to meet their individual needs. We decided that this book should include young people across the spectrum, from preschoolers through young adults, whose families are from all walks of life and are culturally and ethnically diverse.

Throughout the years I have met many parents who have related their experiences to me. When they first suspect that their children are developing differently it ushers in a flood of emotions that can be very difficult to manage, as is the journey to find the answers for their children. After a diagnosis is made, they search for programs that are essential to their children's well-being and progress — they leave no stone unturned. It is a time that can be very lonely for parents. They often say the support of others who have been down this road is very helpful. Parents hope that they can rely on the community to support and accept their children.

I told Rick that my husband David penned an expression nearly two decades ago that embodies our commitment at *The Help Group*: "Dignity, hope, opportunity, and love are the birthrights of all children." Those with disabilities or differences are entitled to these birthrights like all children. In our conversation we discussed how significant it is for our communities and our society to recognize the dignity and potential of the children. They are not just defined by a label, they are children first, deserving of our respect and acceptance. We talked about how important it is to help spread the message that autism is only a part but not the essence of who they are. They are children to be valued whose worth we must support in every way that we can. As autism awareness continues to grow, the doors of understanding and acceptance will continue to open.

I suggested that in addition to the photos it might be meaningful to accompany the images of the children with the words of their parents and, in some cases, with the words of some of our young people themselves. I would let the parents know that we are looking beyond autism to explore what they want to tell the world about their children, about special moments they have had together, and how they want the world to see their children.

We called a few parents to gauge their willingness to contribute and they were eager to participate in a book that celebrates their children. They were very open to share their thoughts and feelings with me. Having met many of them face to face, it was an unforgettable experience to hear from 45 parents and three young people on the spectrum who spoke for themselves. I feel privileged that they entrusted me with including some of their insights in this book.

And so began *Faces of Promise* — a labor of love of all involved that would be given momentum by remarkable children, adolescents and young adults. Each young person portrayed in this book is unique, but all possess dignity, beauty and promise.

It has been a very moving experience that Rick and I would like to share with you.

Barbara Firestone, Ph.D.

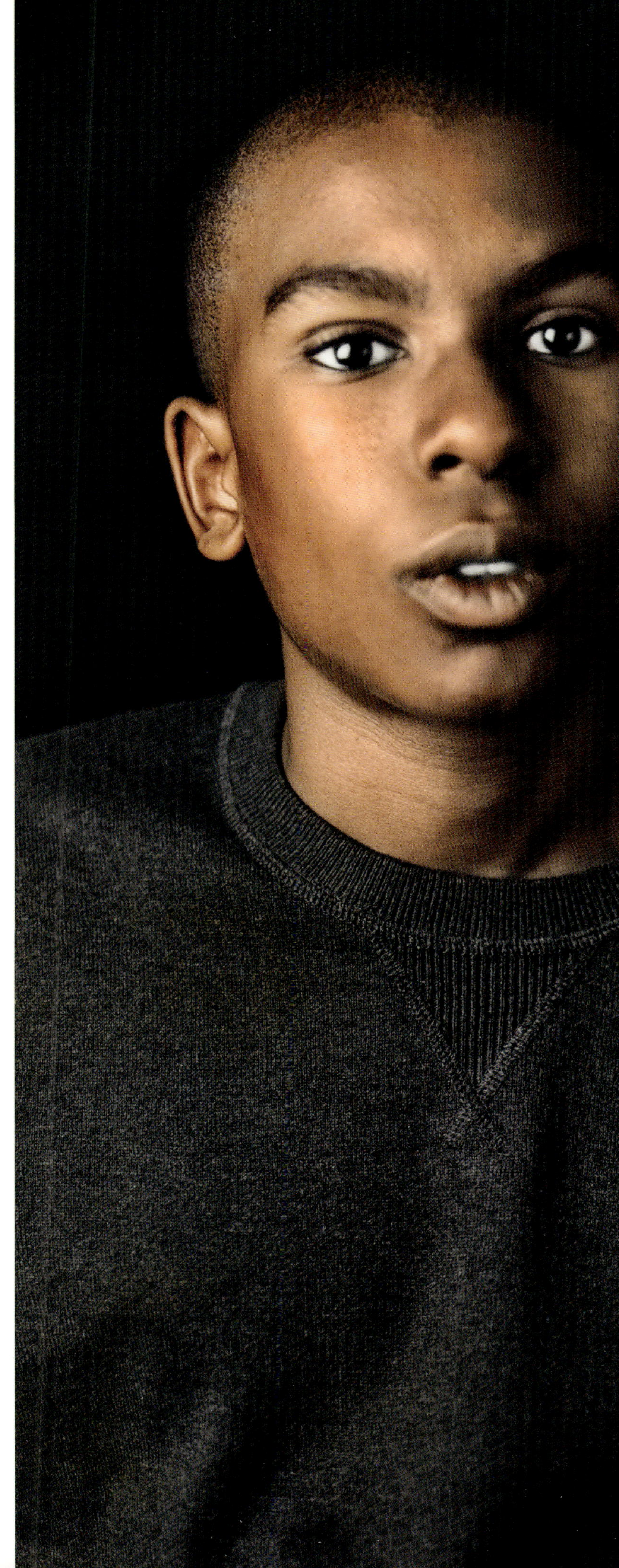

Contents

Ryan	The Help Group	14
Andres	The Help Group	16
Josue & Sebastian	The Help Group	18
Kyler	The Help Group	20
Kaden	The Help Group	22
Rachel	The Help Group	24
Ocean & DuShore	The Help Group	26
Damian	The Help Group	28
Vera	The Help Group	30
Elijah	The Help Group	32
Fionna	The Help Group	34
Romir	The Bay School	36
Tindra & Aeris	The Help Group	38
Lathan	The Help Group	40
Muhammed	The Bay School	42
Tevin	The Help Group	44
Racquel	The Bay School	46
Jimmy	The Help Group	48
Abigail	The Help Group	50
Michael	The Help Group	52
Henry	The Bay School	54
Rakim	The Help Group	56
Pablo	The Bay School	58
Sean & Molly	The Bay School	60
Kasten	The Bay School	62
Christopher	The Bay School	64
Gabe	The Bay School	66
Nicholas	The Help Group	68
Britney & Adrian	The Help Group	70
Thaddeus	The Help Group	72
Chester	The Help Group	74
Cullen	The Help Group	76
Jaz	The Help Group	78
Ben	The Help Group	80
Savanna	The Bay School	82
Tali	The Help Group	84
Alex	The Help Group	86
Kenneth & Daniel	The Help Group	88
A Few Closing Thoughts		90
With Our Special Thanks		91
The Help Group		92
The Bay School		95
About Autism		96
Biographies		98
Acknowledgments		100
20"x24" Polaroid Camera		103

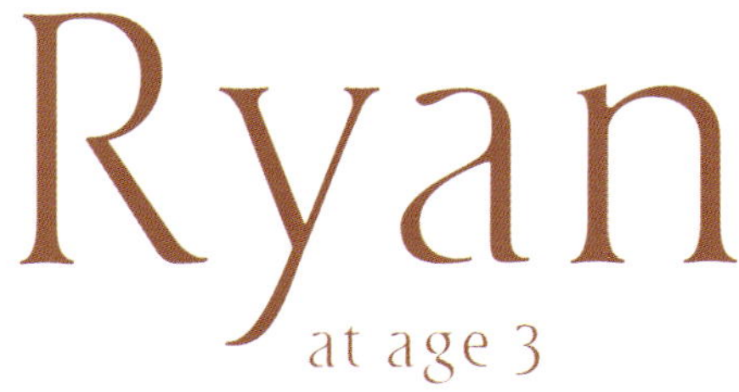

Ryan
at age 3

...a shining light...

Ryan just celebrated his 4th birthday. But in our eyes he has just been born. We have never given up hope and the commitment to love, learn, nurture, teach, support and chip away at Ryan's wall.

We now see a shining light and joy to be shared with others along Ryan's journey. We are so appreciative for those people who have dedicated their life's work to help, encourage and support the children, adults and families who are touched with autism.

~Patrick, Ryan's father

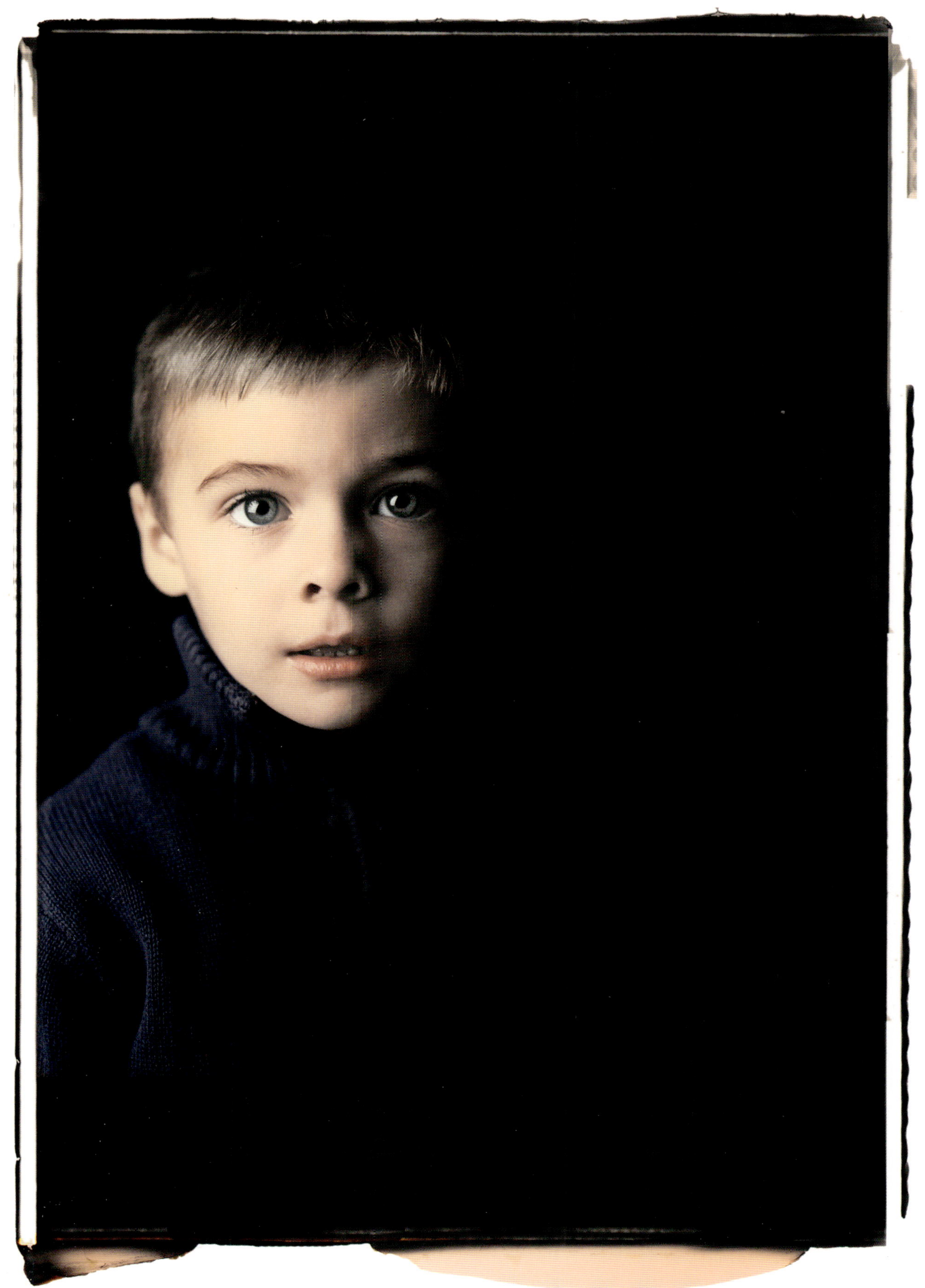

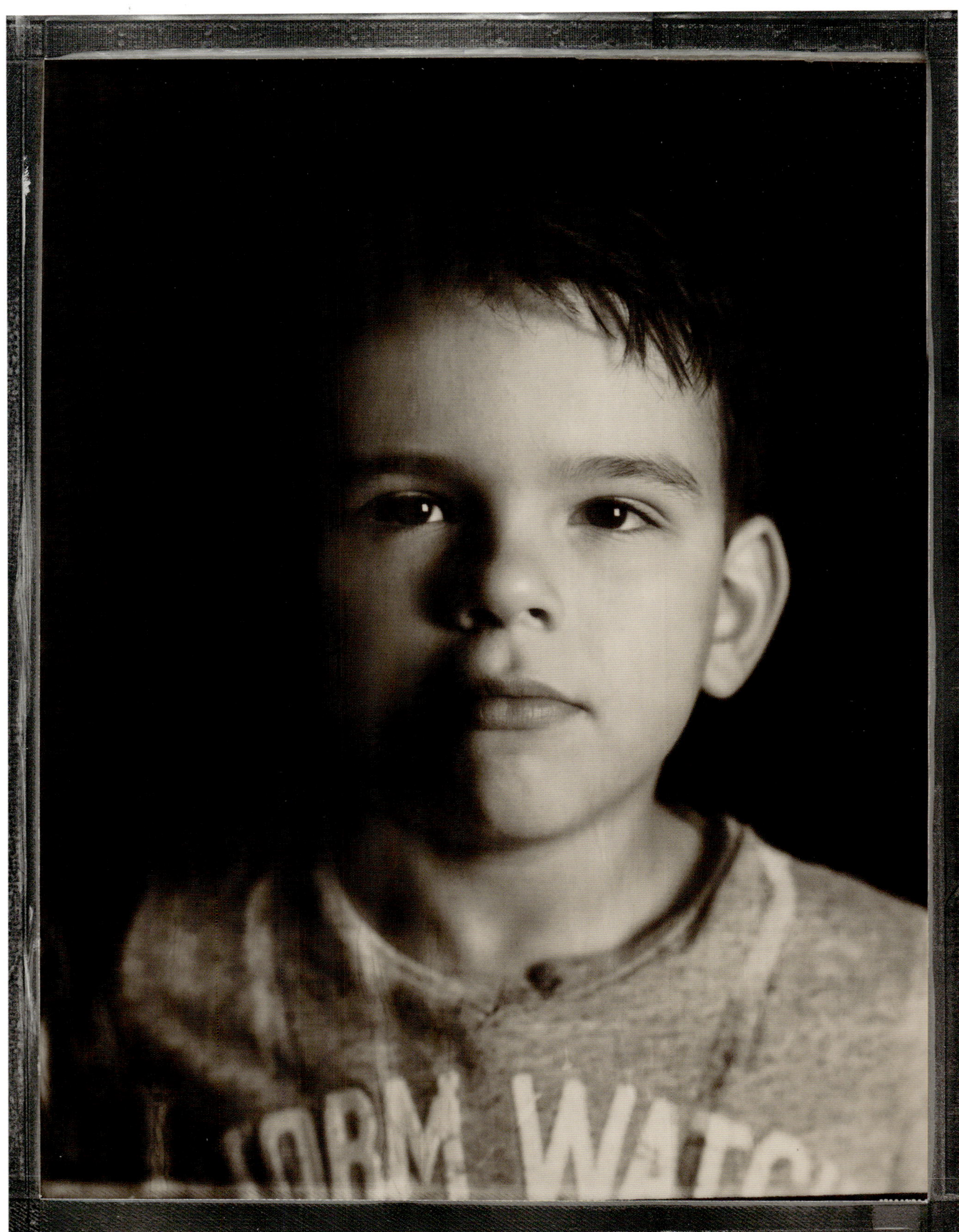
ORM WAT

Andres

at age 4

...the little things.

I forget sometimes that Andres has autism. It's just part of who he is and he's just wonderful. You've just got to get to know him, got to kind of dance with him. And he's great. He makes me a better person.

It's the simple things. Like in the morning, we watch Curious George before going to school. He has breakfast and he jumps on my chair and just sits with me. He's got a great sense of humor too, and he loves laughing. It's just in general, the little things.

~Ricardo, Andres's father

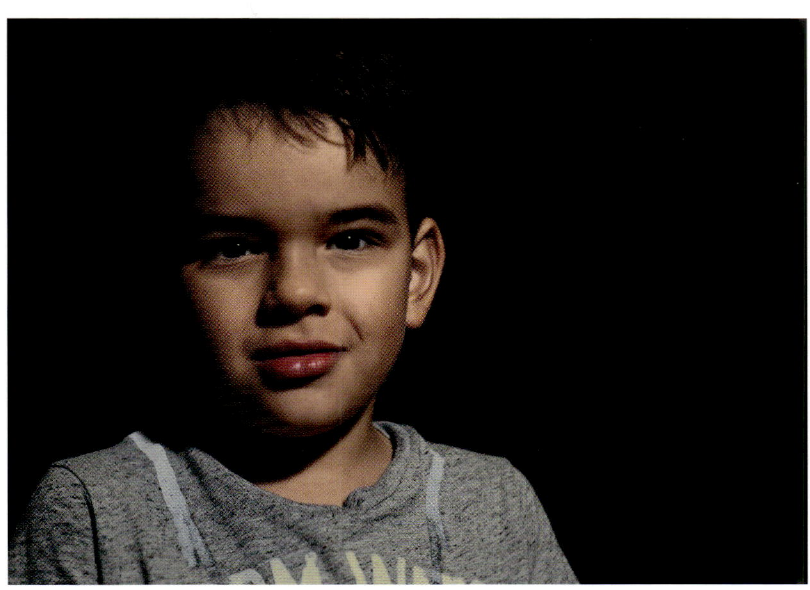

Josue & Sebastian

...it's very beautiful.

At first, Josue did not speak much and I noticed that he hardly understood anything by the age of two. When he started school, he began to understand more, talk more, and the moment came when he hugged me, and said to me, 'Love Mommy.' I cried. I was waiting a long time for that moment.

Every day when Sebastian would come home I would ask him, 'How was school?' And he wouldn't even look at me. Then one day, after a while, I asked him, 'How was school?' and he replied, 'Good.' He also hugged me and sa d, 'I love you.' One thinks that moment will never arrive and all of a sudden, it arrives, and it's very beautiful.

~Rosario, Josue's and Sebastian's mother, translated from Spanish

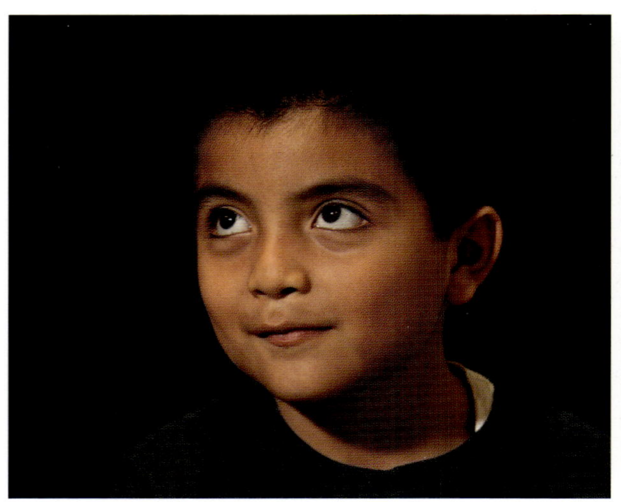
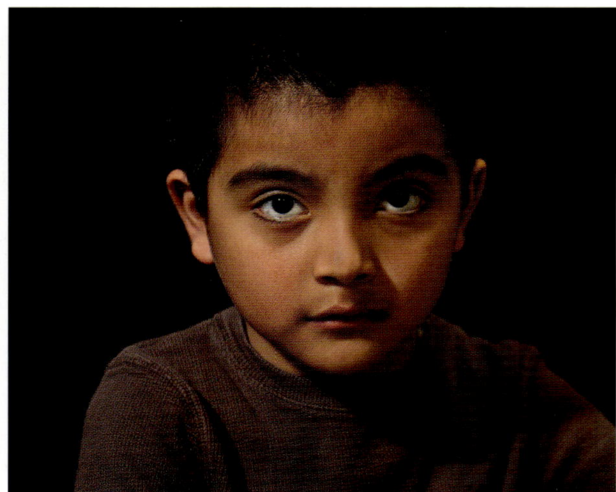
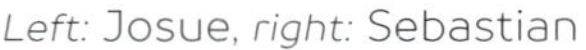

Left: Josue, *right:* Sebastian

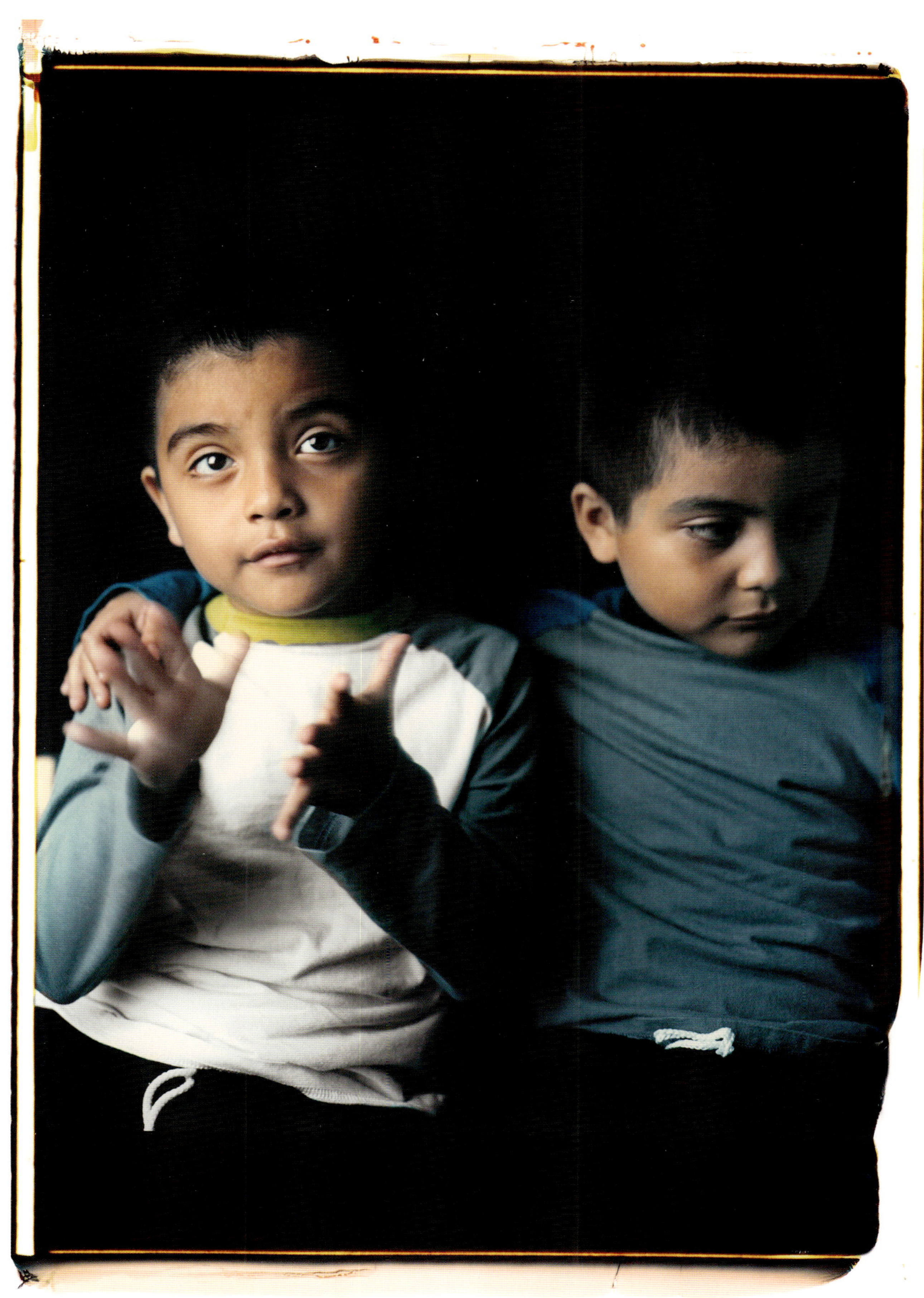

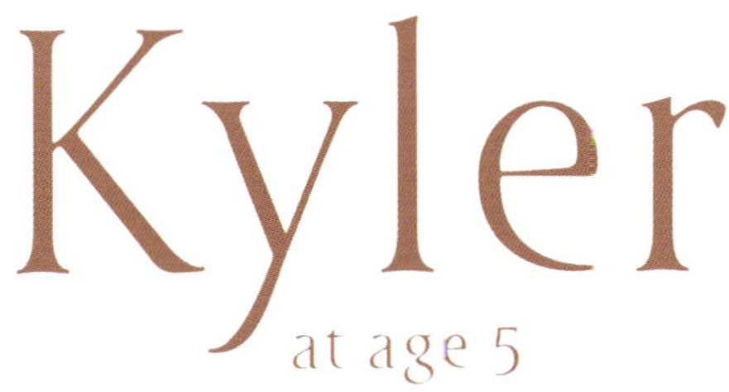

Kyler

at age 5

...it was amazing.

Kyler is such a talented, active, energetic kid. The Special Olympics World Games event was something that we'll never forget. For Kyler, he was able to showcase his skills. It made us open our eyes to the possibilities of what he can achieve.

~Charles, Kyler's stepfather

For him to have the opportunity to go onto the balance beam and the bars, it was amazing. If he's not offered or provided an opportunity, there's no way for him to explore or to experience things or possibilities of what he can achieve. So having that opportunity given to him is very vital.

~Jocelyn, Kyler's mother

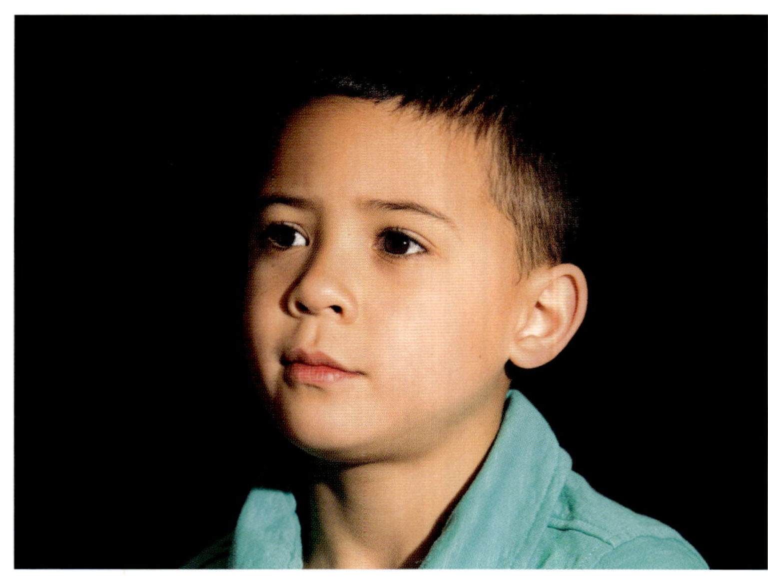

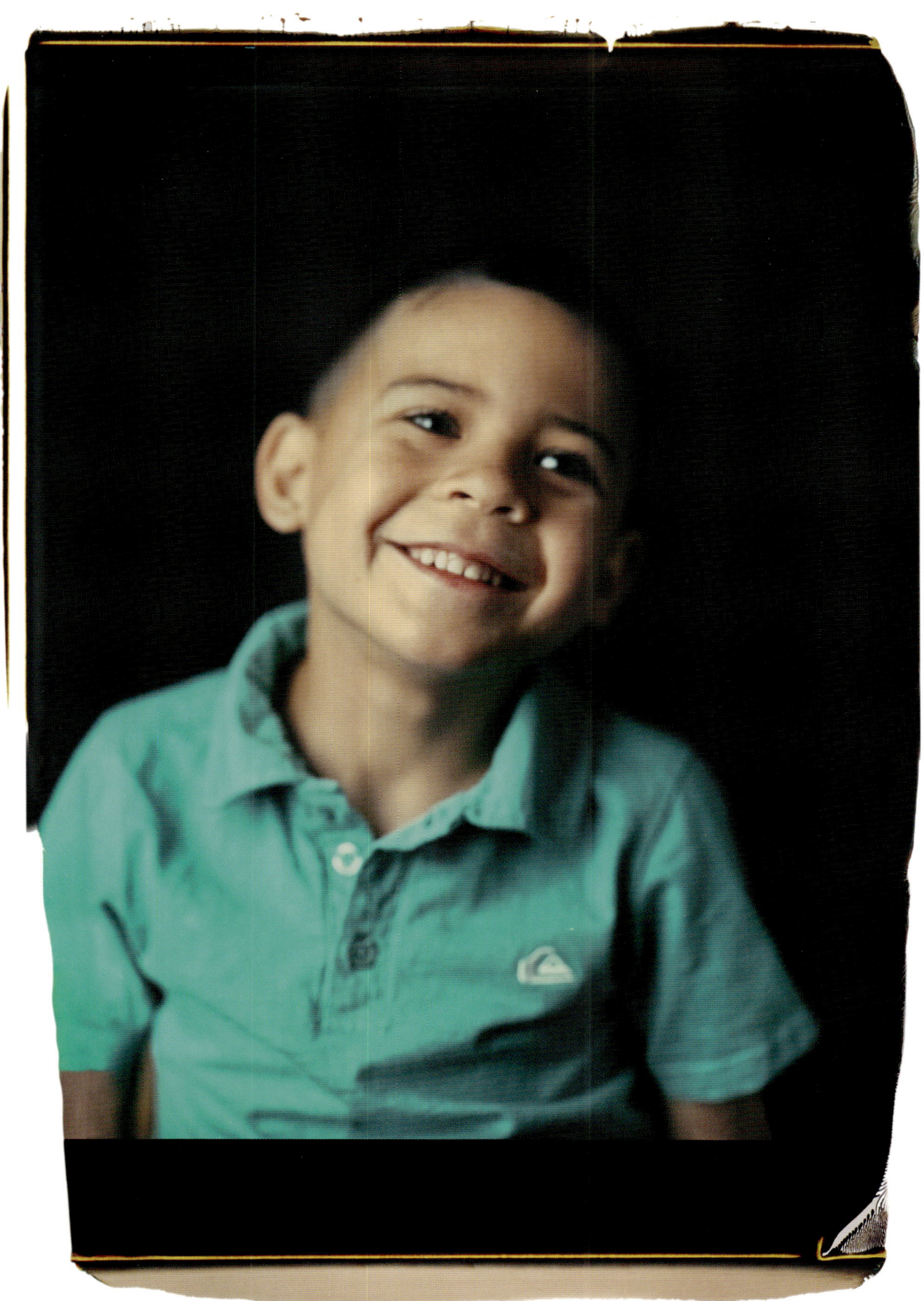

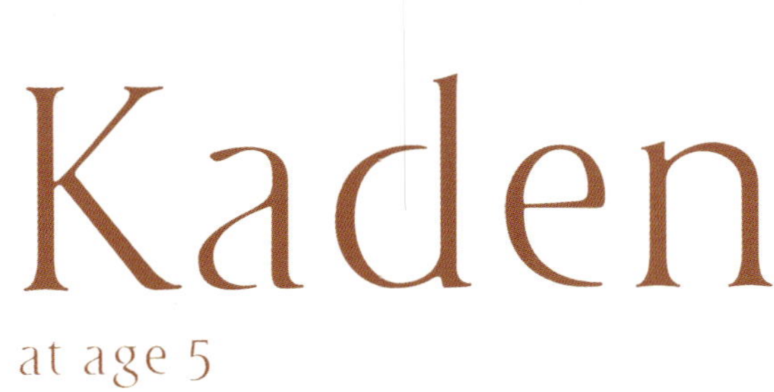

Kaden
at age 5

He's my everything.

A very special moment for me was when I gave birth to Kaden and saw his little face. Just being with Kaden is a special moment. He's my everything. He's my life. If he's happy, I'm happy. Kaden is happiest when he's jumping on a trampoline, or running, or playing chase with daddy.

~Patricia, Kaden's mother

As adults, life can weigh things down, but to be in the moment — Kaden is always in the moment. For example, seeing him participate in Christmas last year was great. We took Kaden to an L.A. mall where they have snowfalls during the holidays. When it snowed, he'd look up at it a while sitting atop my shoulders and that was special.

~Jason, Kaden's father

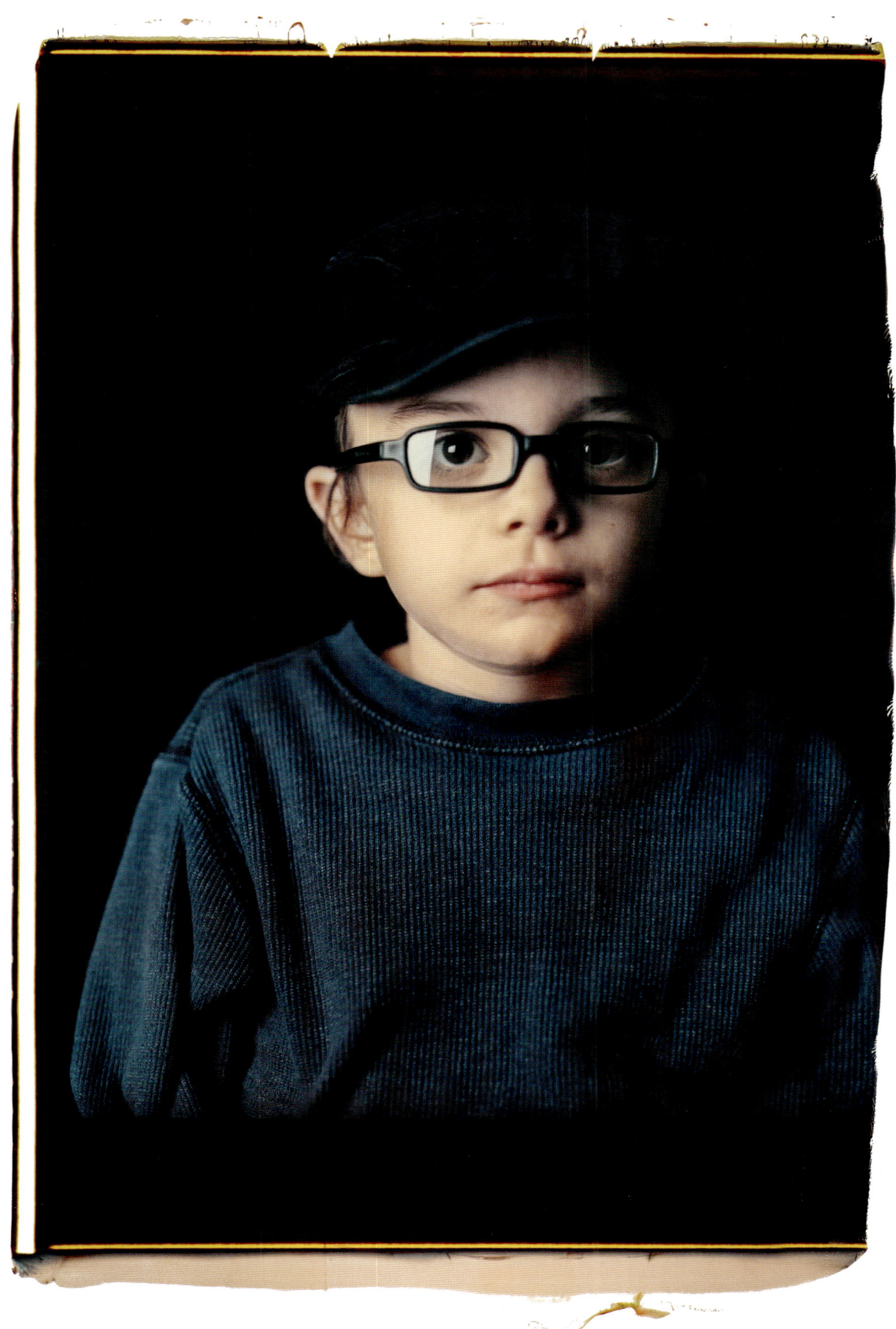

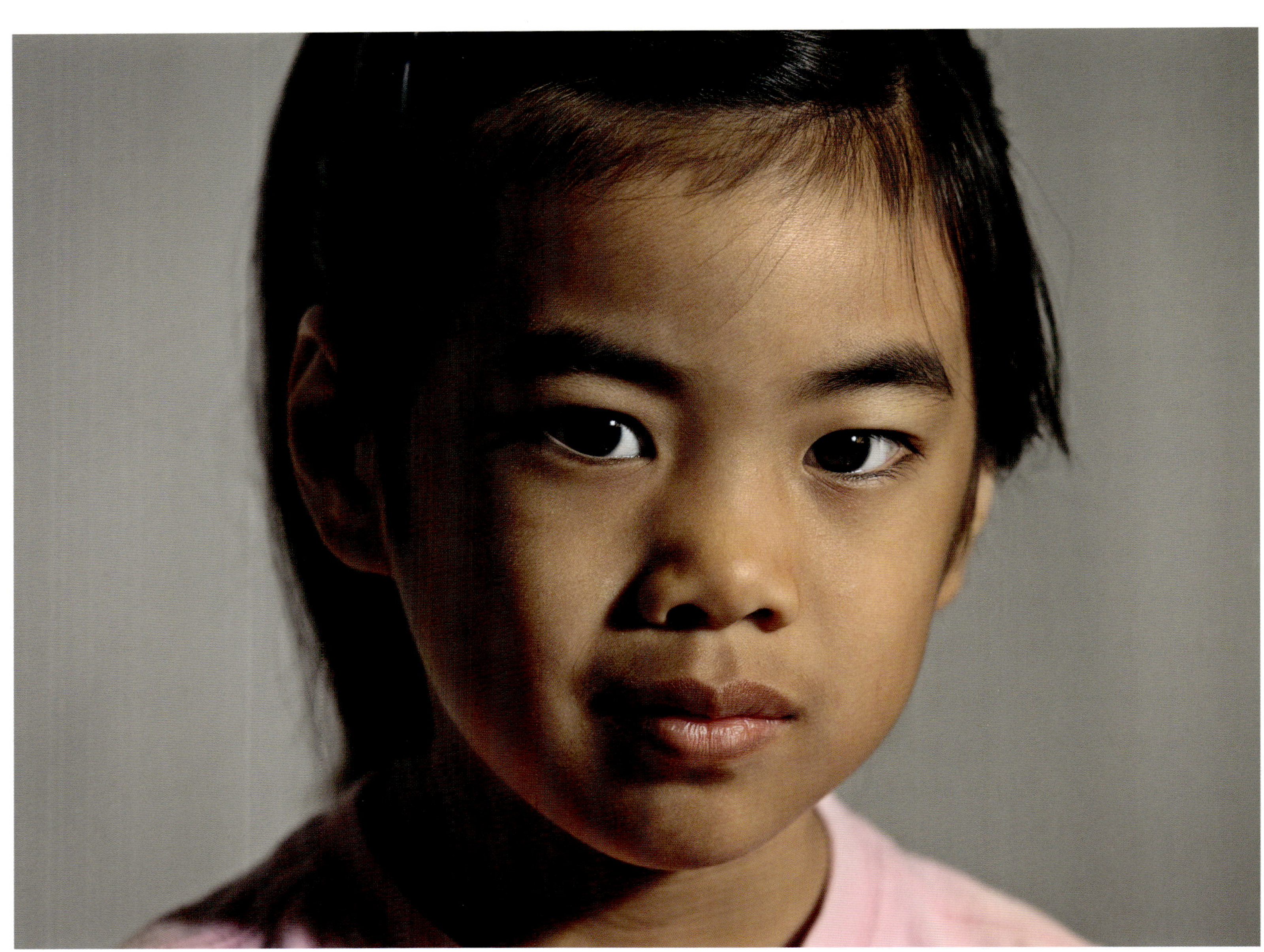

Rachel

...she's getting to know me...

We're very grateful that Rachel can now use some words to communicate her needs to us. When she started school she didn't make any eye contact, or say even one word. So we know she has potential. Like other children with autism, she just needs more help to improve, to make progress.

Three years ago was the first time Rachel started to call me, 'Daddy' and about a year ago, she started to give me hugs. I was very happy. I feel like she's getting to know me, and I'm hoping that our bond will keep growing.

~Tan, Rachel's father

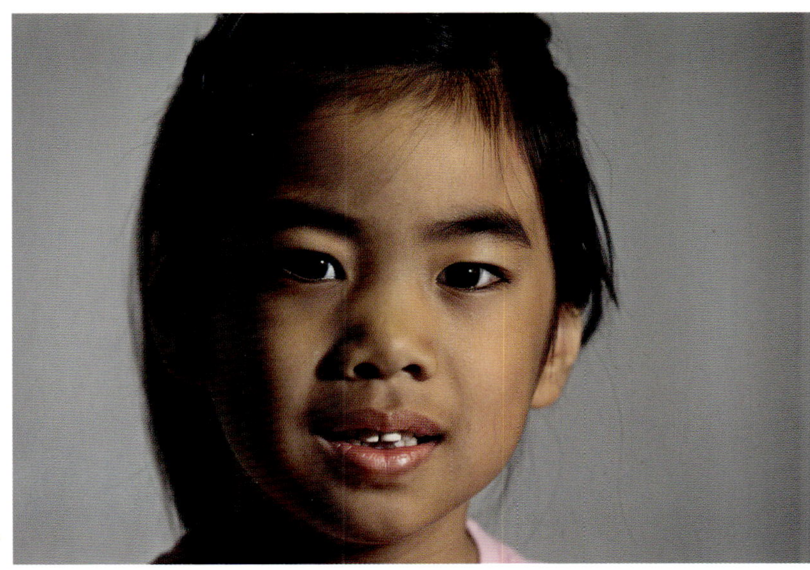

Ocean & DuShore

twin brothers, at age 6

...they deserve acceptance...

My sons and I like to dance. Ocean loves computers, and he knows how to work a laptop better than I do. DuShore loves to sing — singing is his passion. They love going to school. They really enjoy discovering new things out in the world.

I want the world to know that although my boys have autism, they deserve acceptance and understanding just like any other child.

~Sharise, Ocean's and DuShore's mother

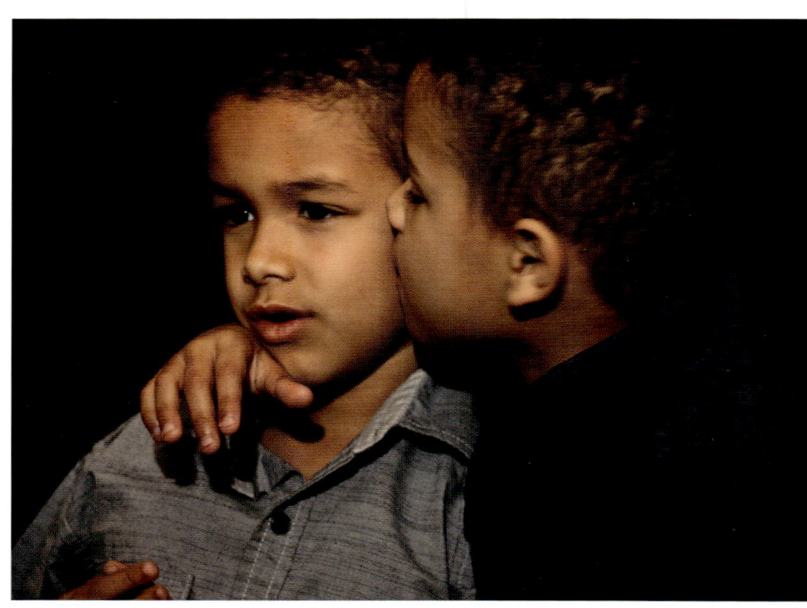

Left: DuShore, *right:* Ocean

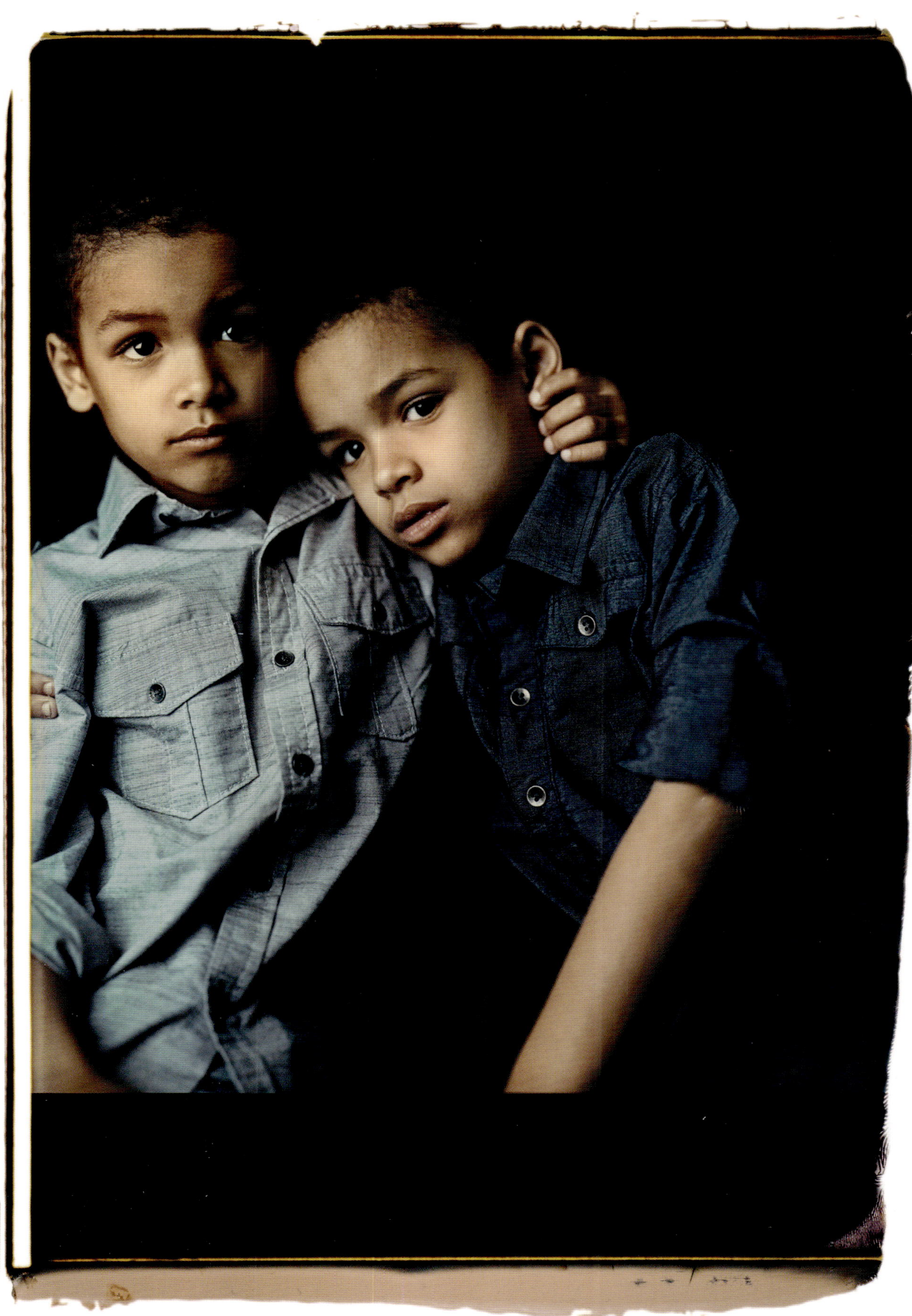

Damian

at age 6

...he's a good kid.

I raise my grandson Damian. I have taught him that he has autism. I've taught him that autism isn't something that should label him, or make him less than others. He can think, reason and feel. And I've taught him how to bring out his feelings.

Damian has lots of wonderful qualities. He moves me a lot of the time. He is always smiling, always laughing with a happy face — he's a good kid.

~Gabriela, Damian's grandmother,
translated from Spanish

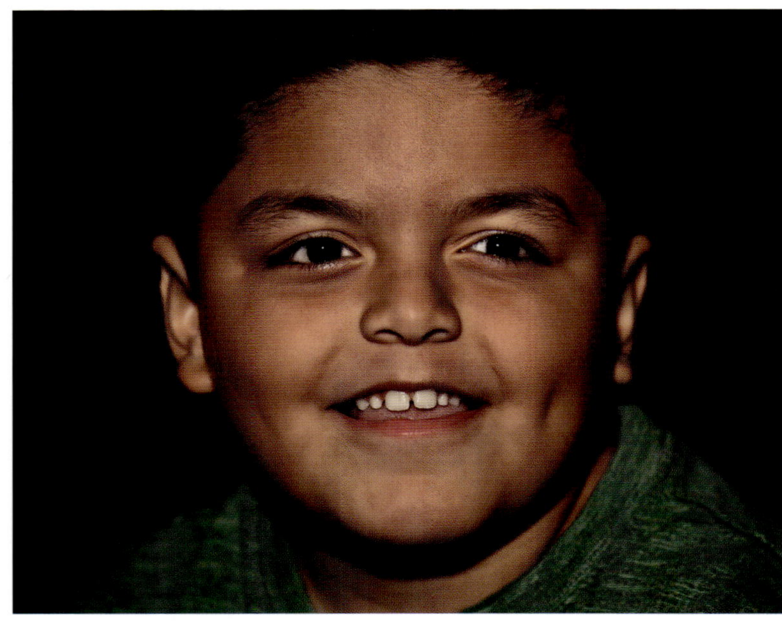

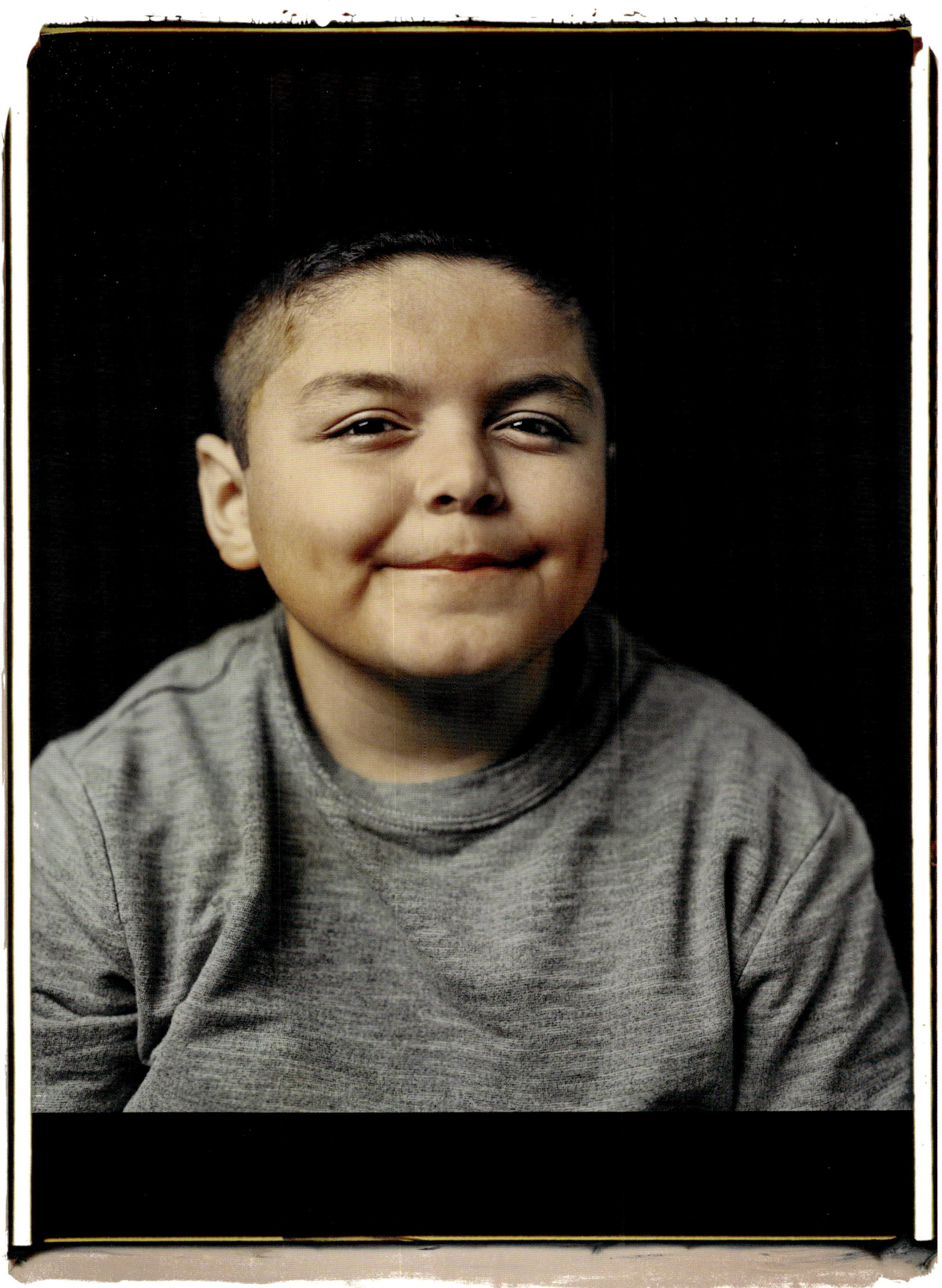

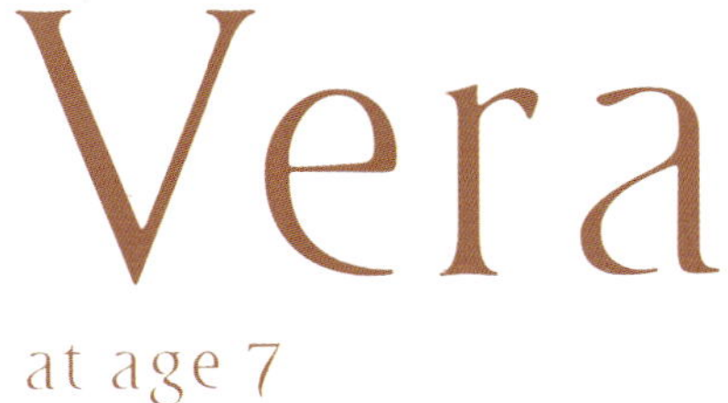

Vera

at age 7

...brighter than the sun.

Every time Vera is successful, we celebrate a happy moment, we celebrate every small task she accomplishes. She feels like she's 10 feet tall. I tell her, 'I know it's in you.' Vera is full of lots of potential.

Vera loves to make music with her dad. When we're all together enjoying the music, Vera is brighter than the sun. She's so happy, she's got a sparkle.

I want Vera to be able to fulfill her dreams, just like anybody else. Anc, as her parents we are there to help her.

~Conny, Vera's mother

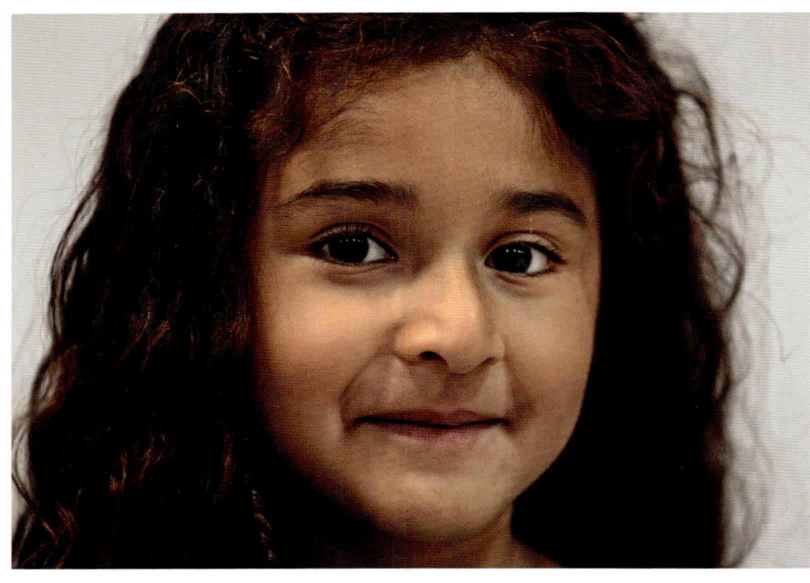

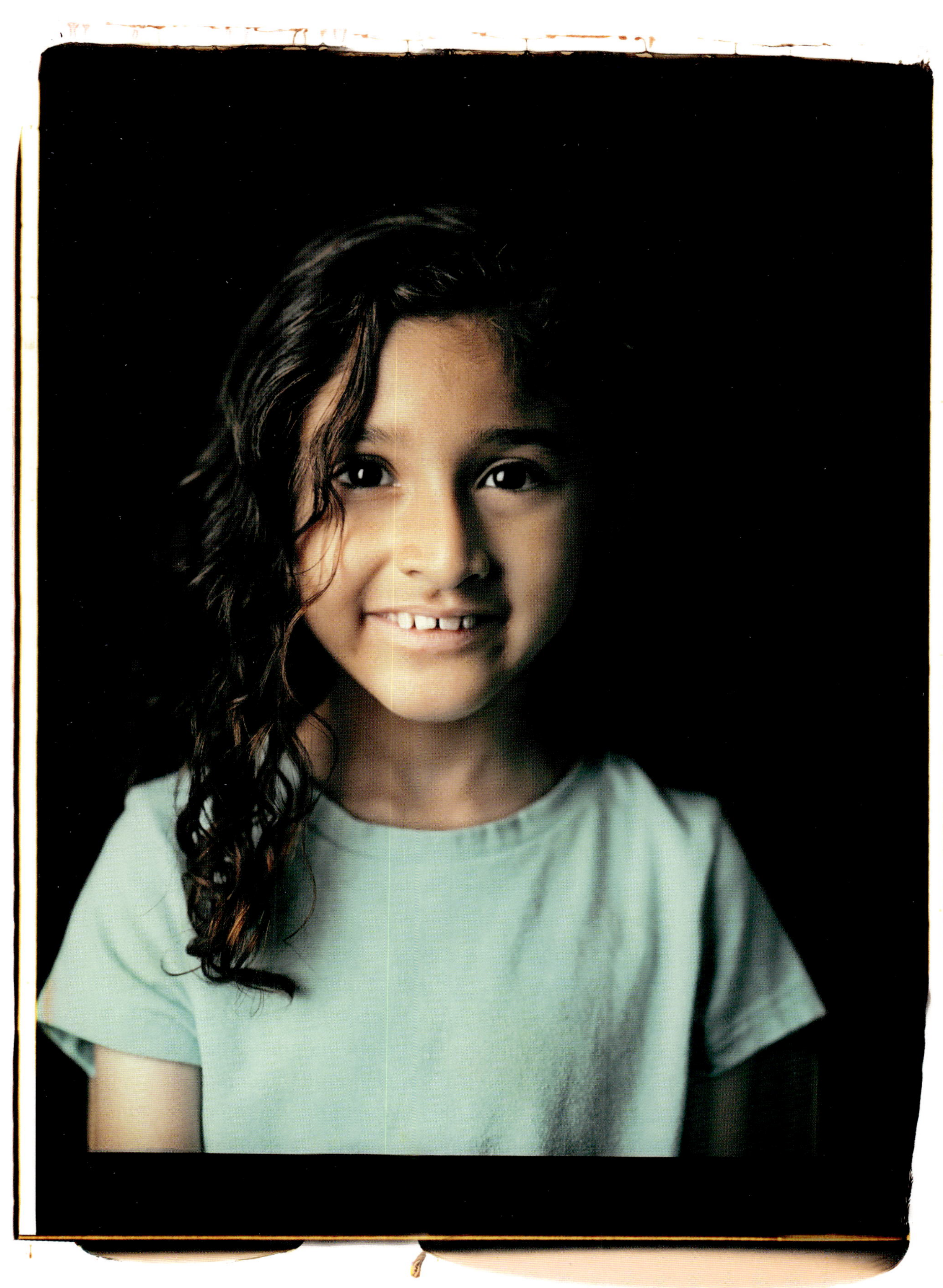

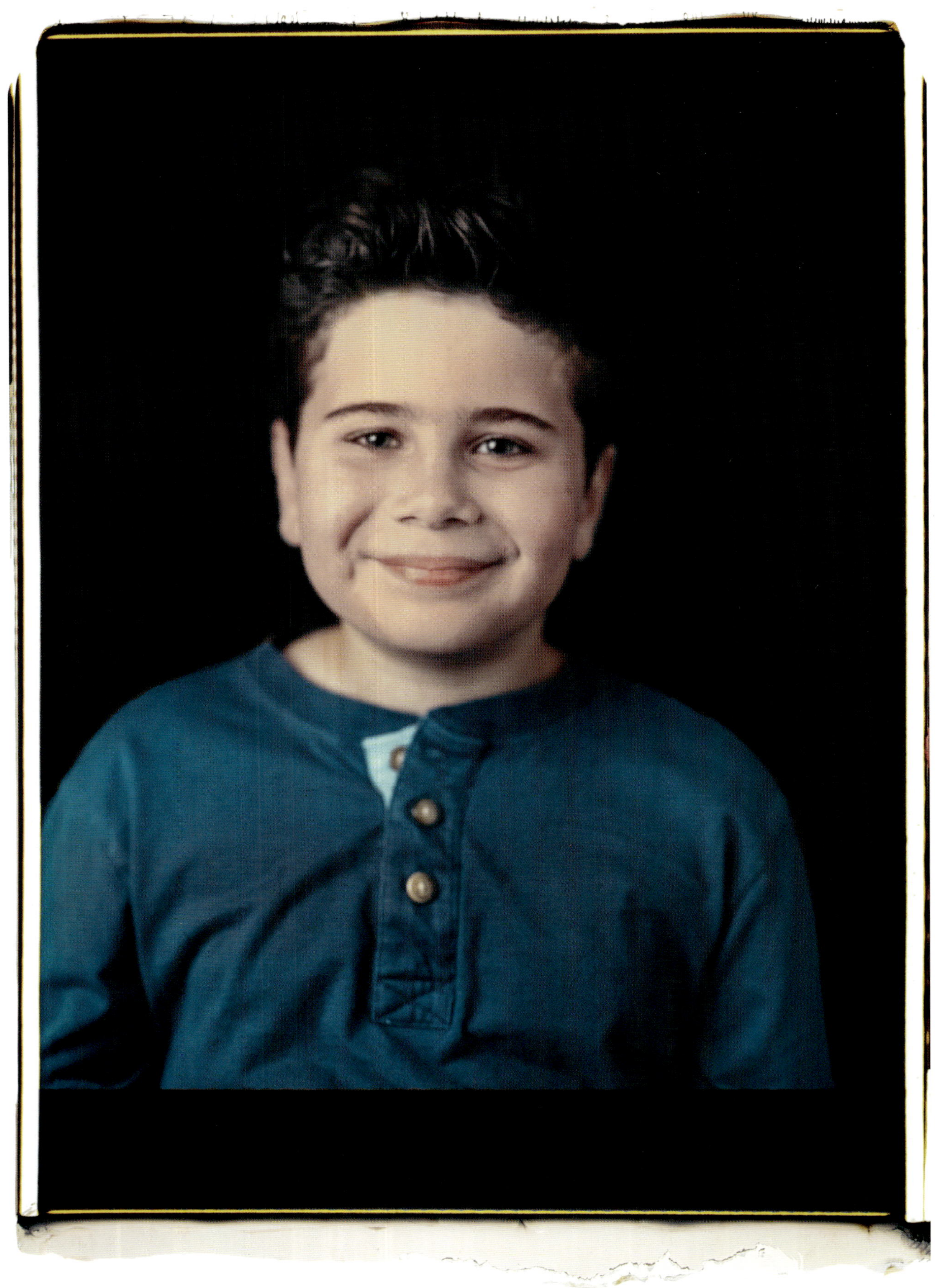

Elijah

...he runs really far.

I hope that Elijah's spark never goes away. I never want to see him
dulled down, or be afraid to try things, or do things. And that's
something I tell him all the time, 'Just try, just try. I'm going to be so
proud of you because you tried. It's not because you won a medal,
or because you got an A, or because you got into the top school or
college. It's you — you're trying.'

Elijah has a light and a brightness. He's able to engage others in his
happiness, his humor, his joy, and his love for life. Now, he's picked up on
things that he's learned, and he's running with it. And he goes, and he
runs really far.

~Anya, Elijah's mother

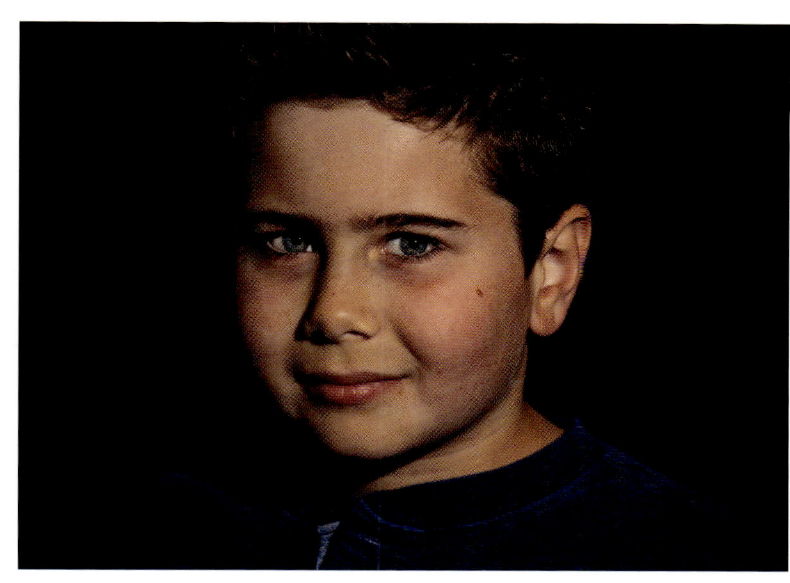

Fionna

at age 7

...to see Fionna happy...

I like to see Fionna happy and smiling. A special time was Fionna's birthday. She was smiling, and gave me a hug without my asking. It's also special when she can shoot the ball into the basket. It makes me happy to see her happy, and able to express this emotion.

It's important to let people know to have more understanding, more acceptance.

~Benny, Fionna's father

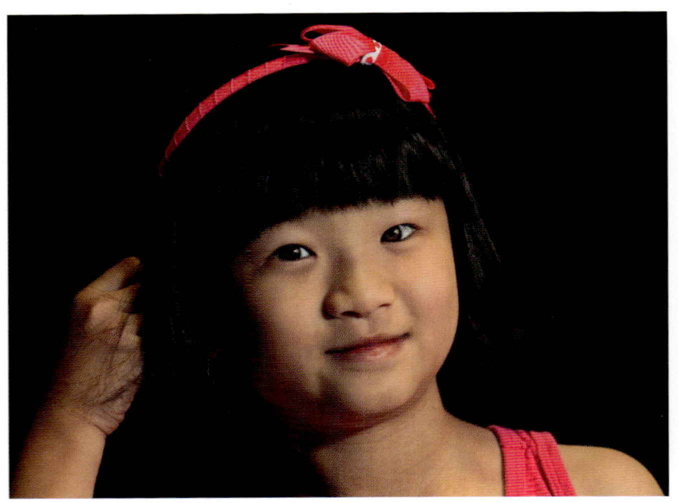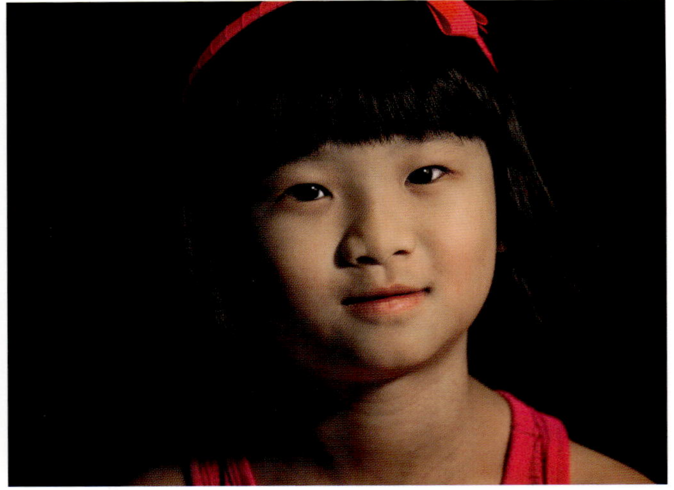

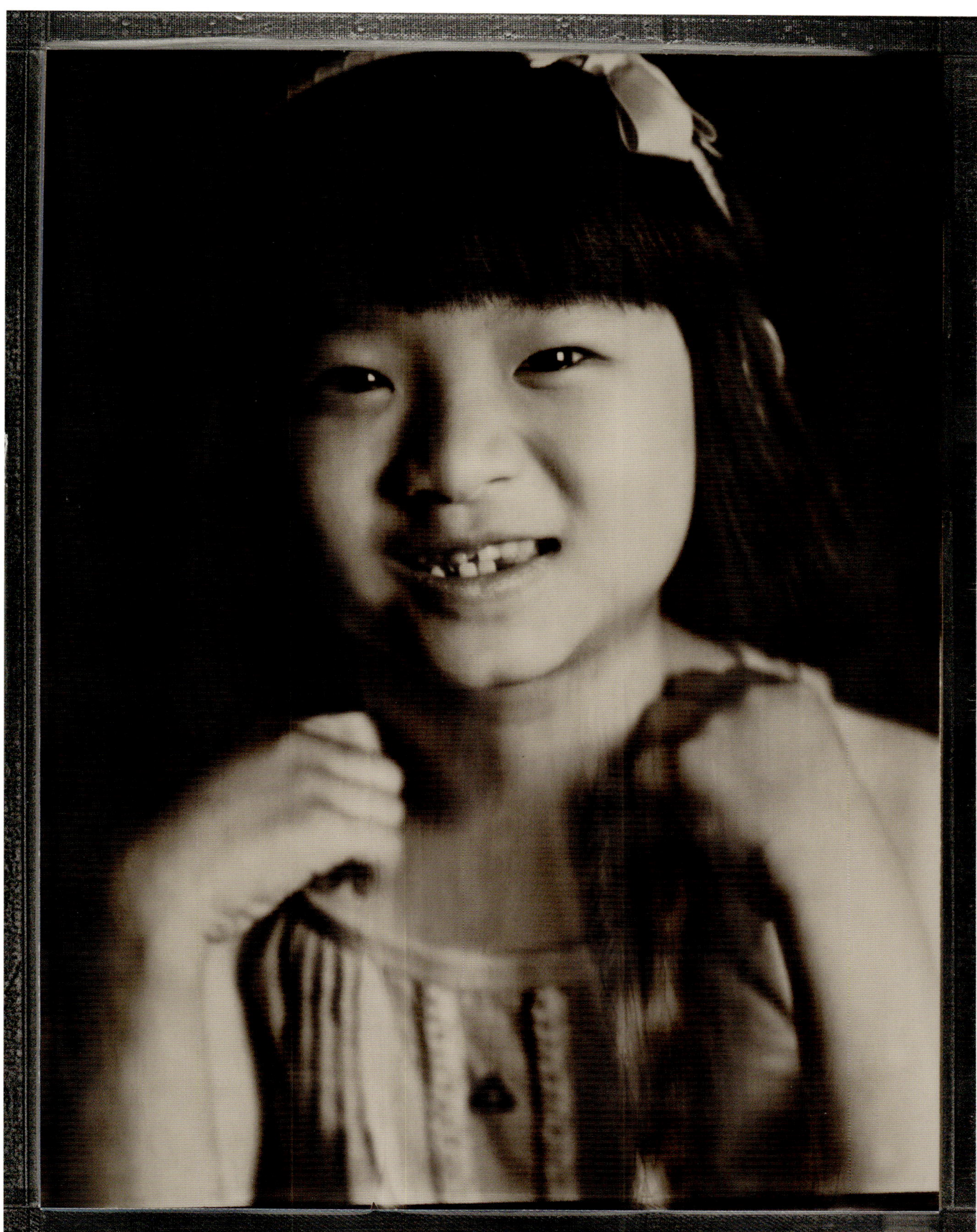

Romir
at age 7

...always in our hearts...

Romir was born on March 5, 2007, and passed away from a heart condition on November 3, 2015, at the tender age of eight. Romir has touched so many lives in such a short span of life.

He was reflective of pure innocence and divinity. He was always smiling. He was so refreshing, he was like a healing balm. Even though Romir was nonverbal, his facial expressions would tell us more than what spoken words are able to. His most joyous moments were going out in the park and swinging in the playground.

Romir is always in our hearts and the moments we have spent with him are the best in our lives.

~Padma and Raj, Romir's parents

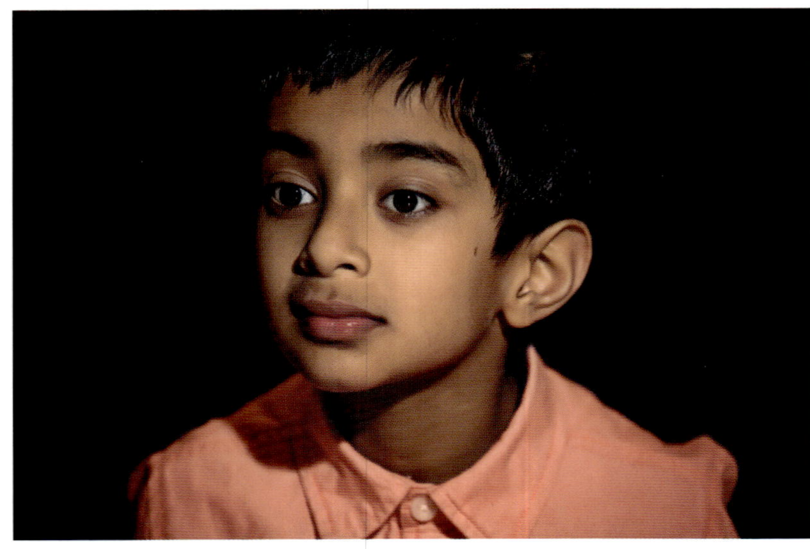

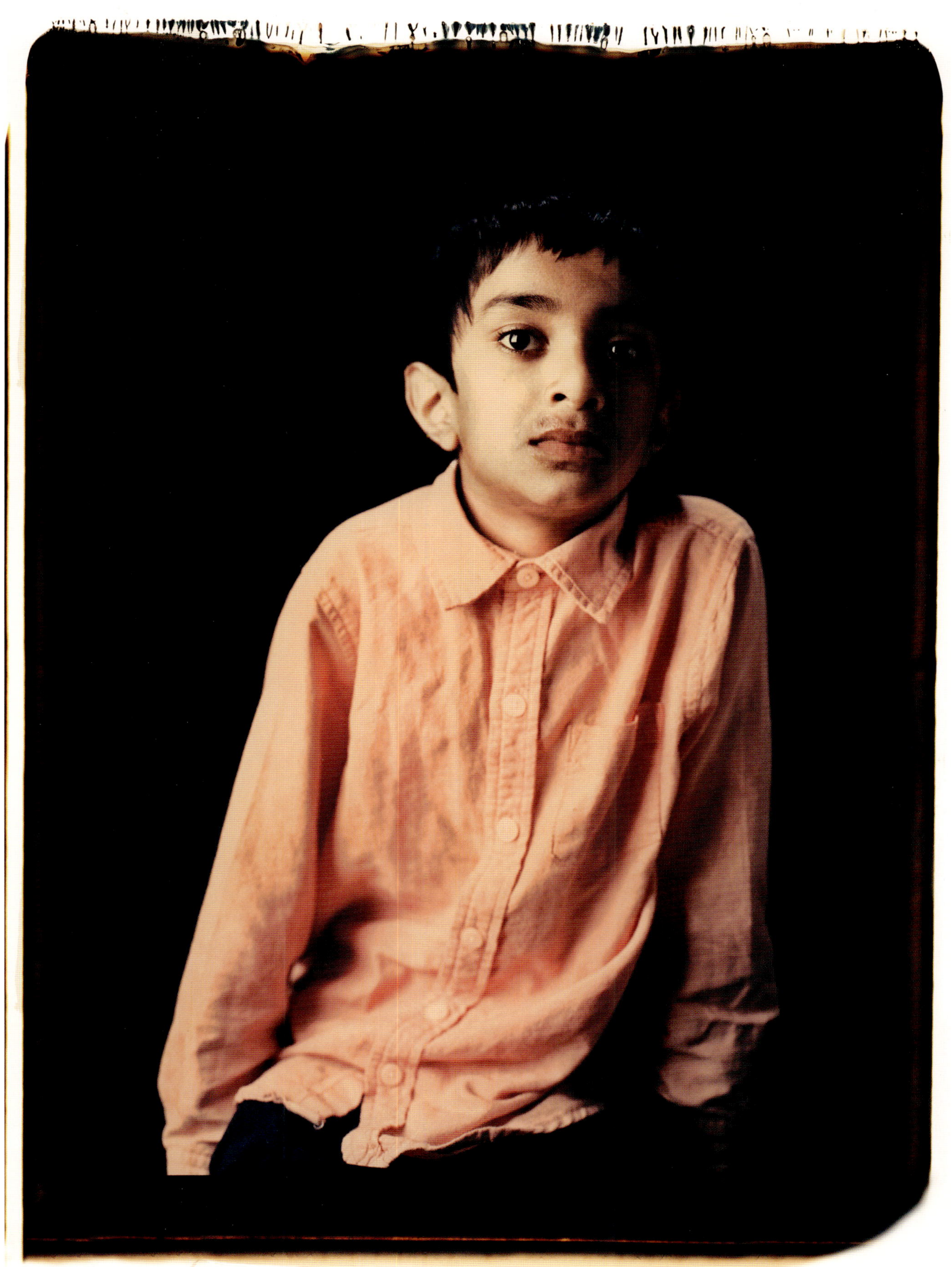

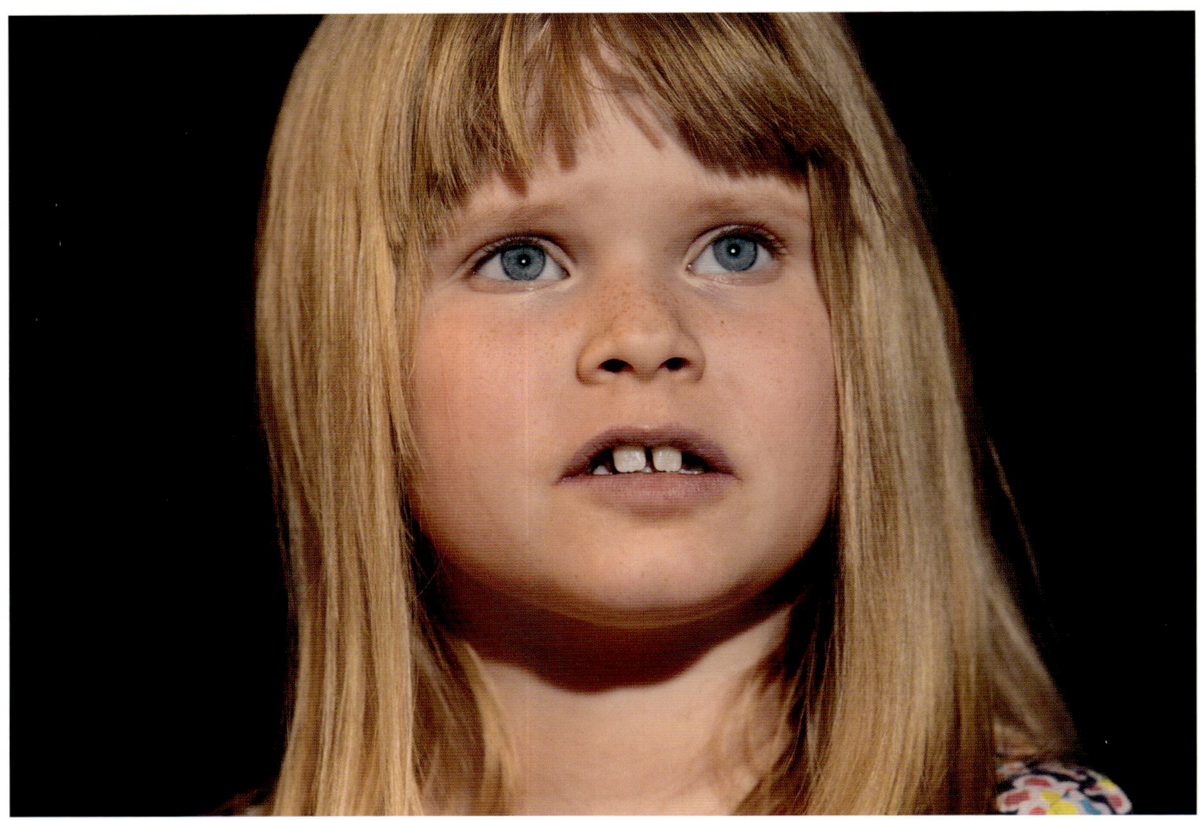

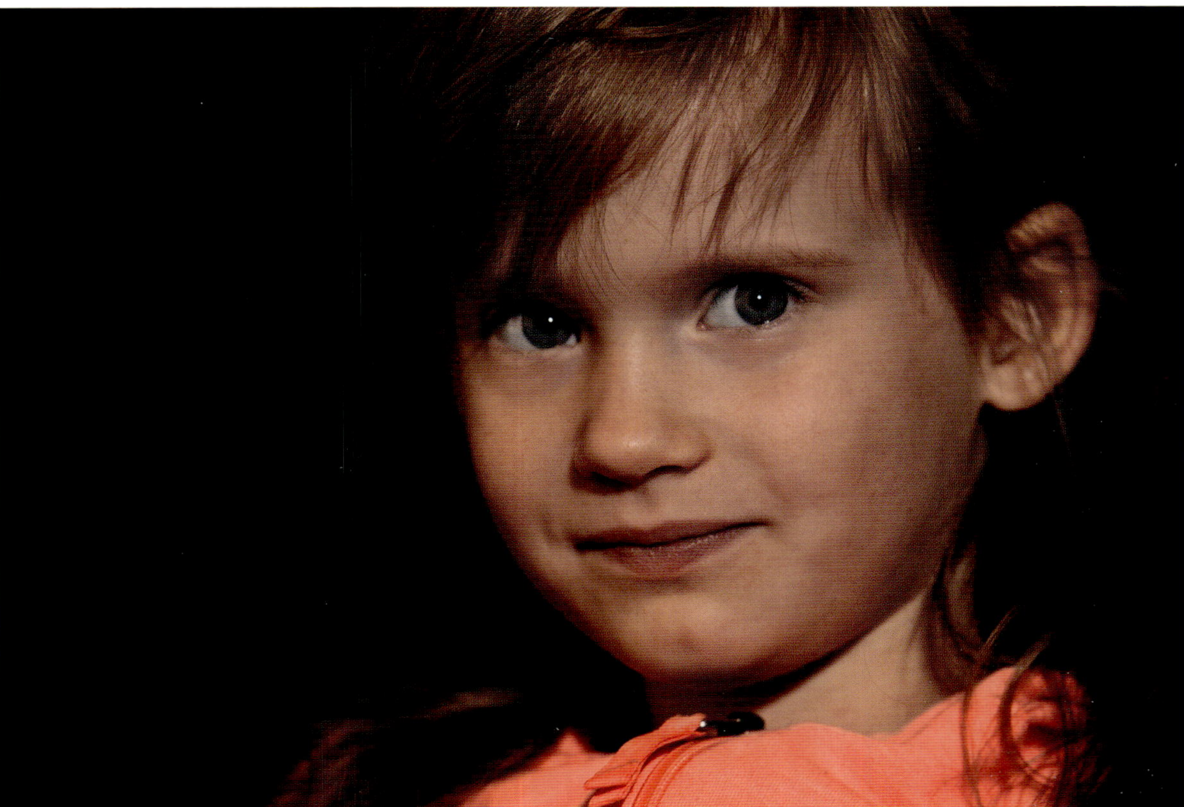

Top: Tindra, *below:* Aeris

Tindra & Aeris

sisters, ages 7 and 5

...I love you mama...

One day in Tindra's room, when we were playing with her toys, we held
a conversation for ten minutes. I was surprised because it has been
difficult for Tindra to have a conversation. She was talking to me, she
was right there in the moment, and we talked about school, her toys,
her siblings and her favorite songs and colors.

Every night I blow the girls kisses and I sing a Swedish lullaby. I started
singing and Aeris sang along every single word even though she doesn't
know what it means, but she knew the melody. After that, she said,
'I love you mama' and the tears came. That was very special.

~Mia, Tindra's and Aeris's mother

Lathan

at age 8

...it's how his heart is.

When I was pregnant with Lathan, *I Hope You Dance* came on the radio and I could not stop crying. I would think about when he was going to be an adult and him getting married and dancing with him.

A couple of months ago he was sitting at the kitchen table with his computer and the song came on, so I told him the story. And all of a sudden he stands up from the table and he says, 'Mom I'm going to make your dream come true.' And he walks over to me, takes my hand and slow dances the entire song in the kitchen with me. It was just one of those moments that I will carry with me forever because it was just so beautiful and sweet — it's how his heart is.

~Laura, Lathan's mother

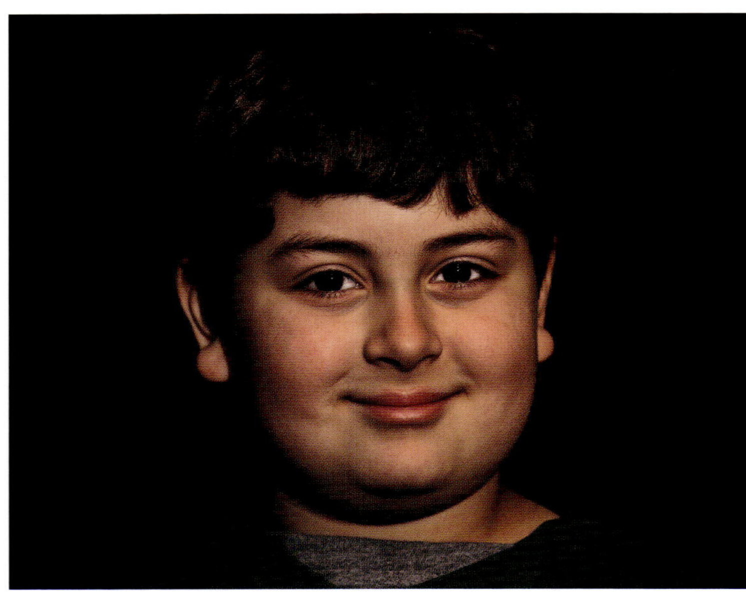

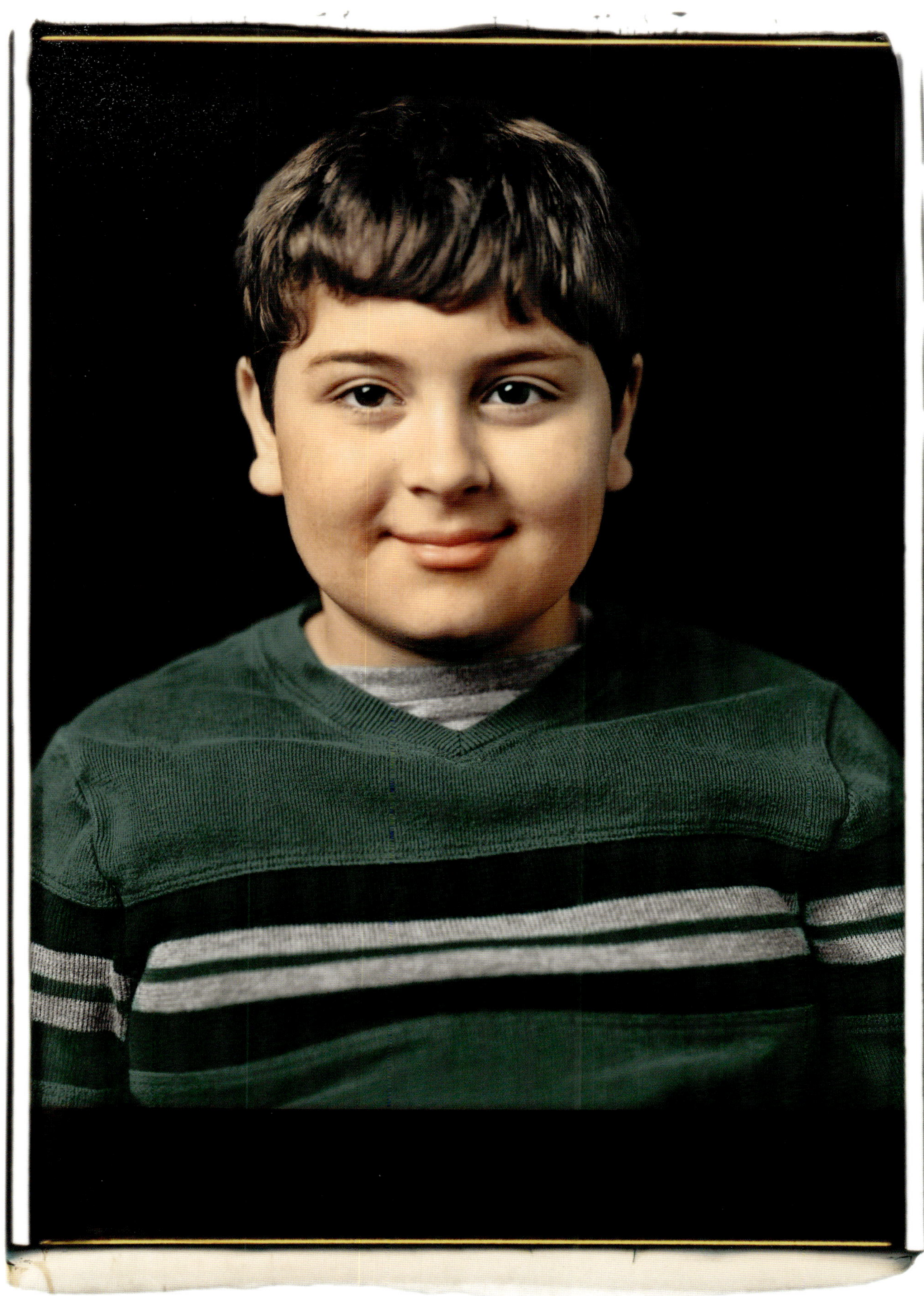

Muhammed

at age 11

He likes to be around people.

Muhammed is happiest when he's out in the community. He loves to hike trails, go to farmers markets, and we are always on the lookout for food and cultural festivals. Some people have the idea that kids with autism may not be social, but Muhammed is the opposite of that. He likes to be around people.

Muhammed likes good food, good music and good people. He is just like everyone else and should be treated that way. I want people to value, to understand and to treat my son, Muhammed, with dignity.

~Feda, Muhammed's mother

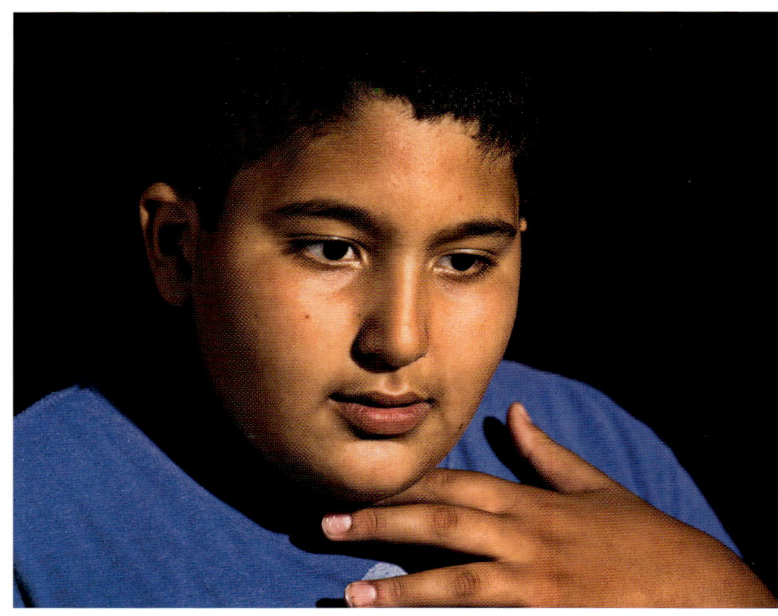

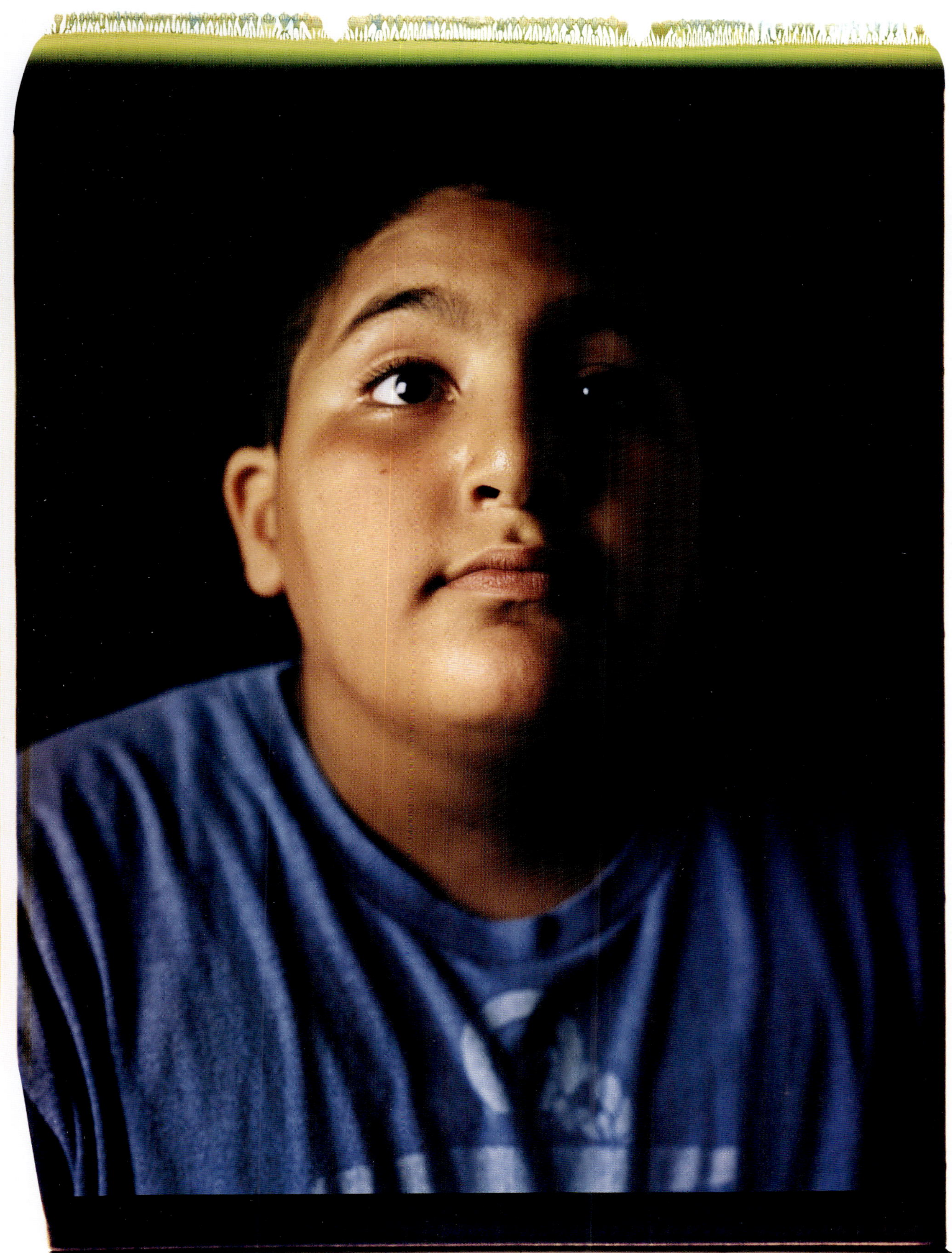

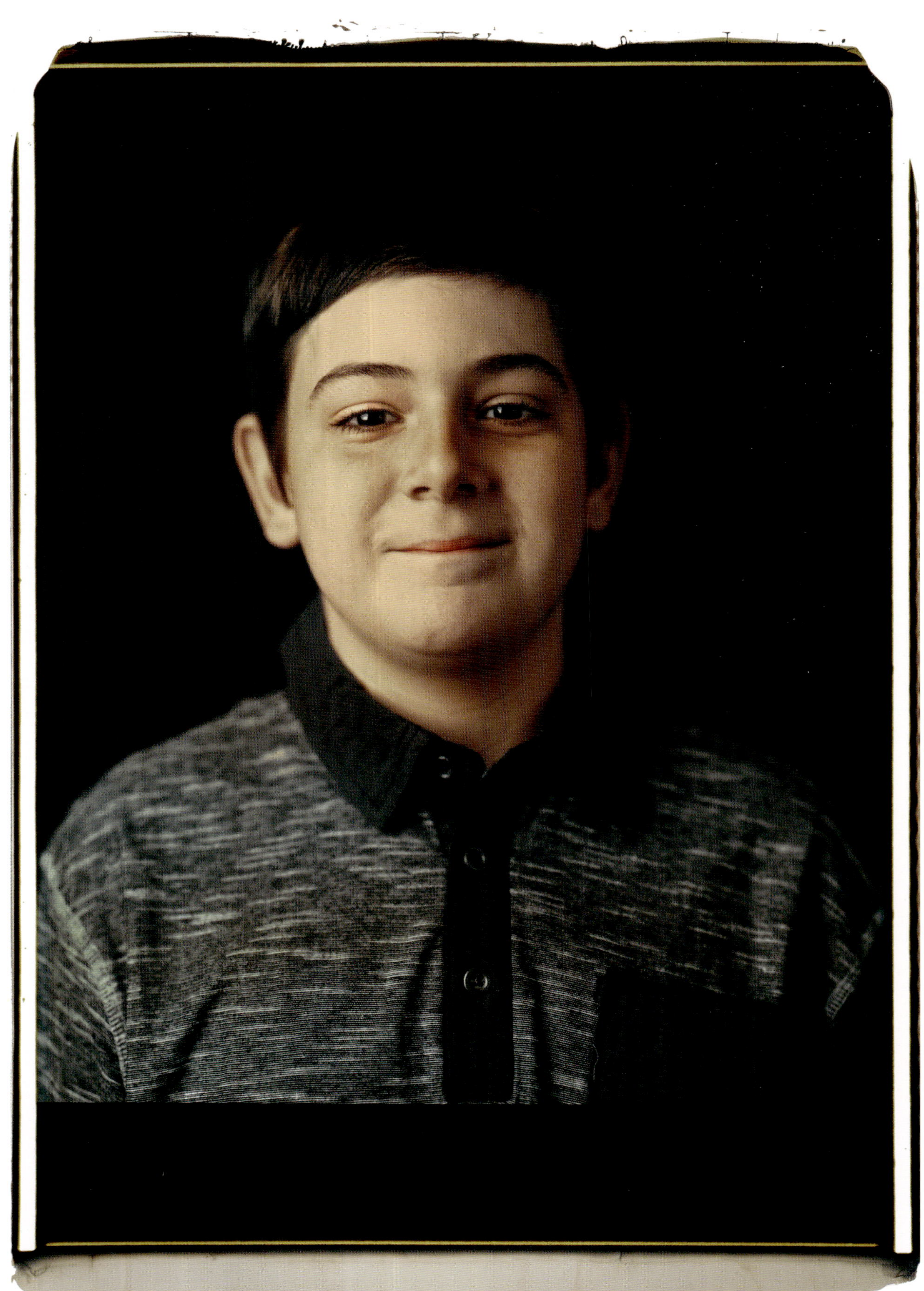

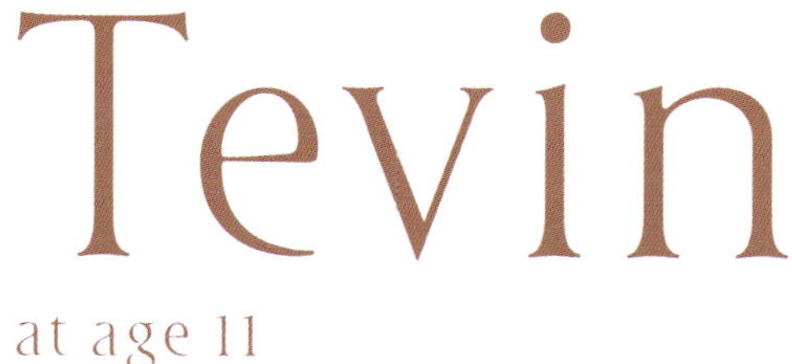

Tevin

It's the best feeling...

There's a lot of things that I have overcome that's got me to here, and it's just been a long journey. I didn't really have a lot of friends, but when I came to my new school I made a lot of friends.

I'm proud of my skills that I'm going to use as an adult to get a job. I want to work on games, maybe programming.

It feels pretty good when I learn new things. It's like, this energy, going on inside of me, making me go, 'Yes'. It's the best feeling you could feel.

~Tevin, in his own words

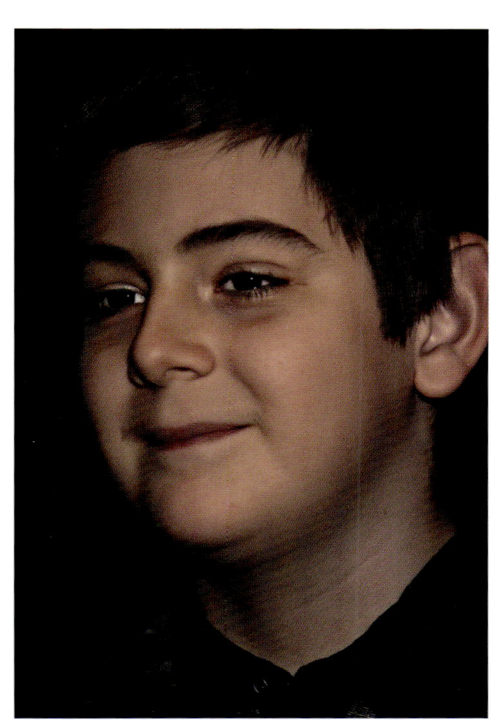

Racquel

at age 11

Our life is always full of surprises...

Our life is always full of surprises with Racquel. When she was in preschool her teacher told us that Racquel knew her colors even though the teacher hadn't taught them yet. When she was six, she was in a ballet recital that I expected to be very challenging for her, but she was considered the superstar. It was such a happy moment for her, she wanted to do it again.

Racquel taught herself how to draw anime. She likes to make earrings. She loves music. She's happy when our family is together. These times that we share have become a special part of me.

~Tess, Racquel's mother

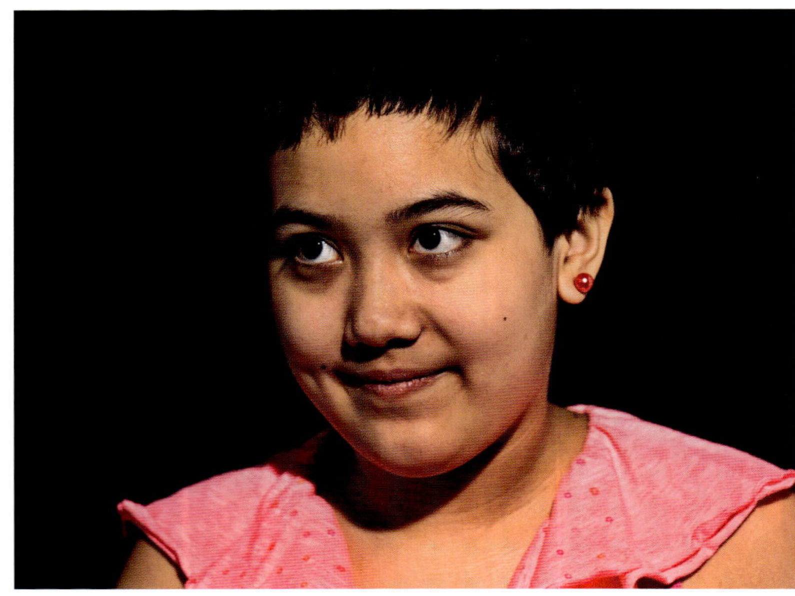

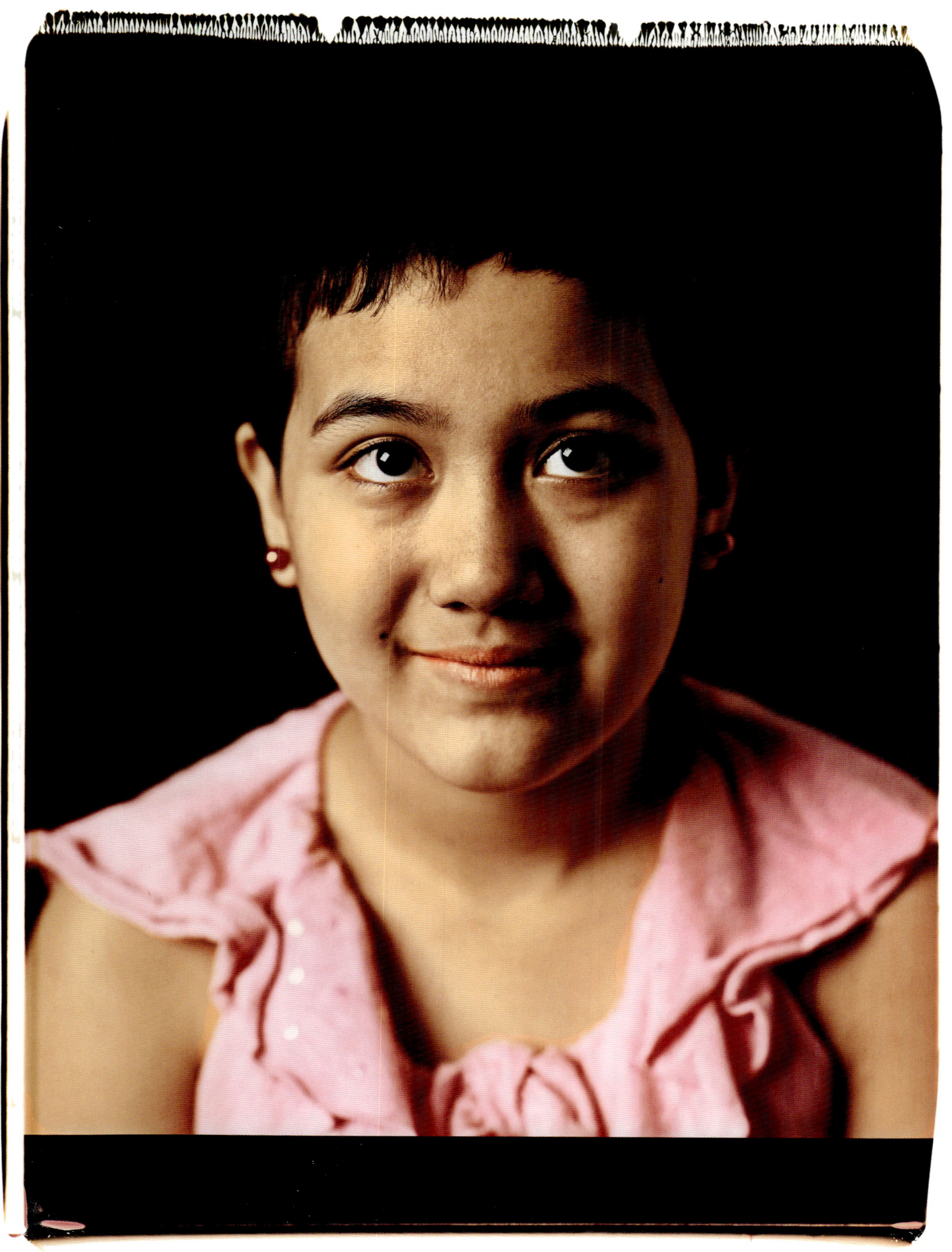

Jimmy

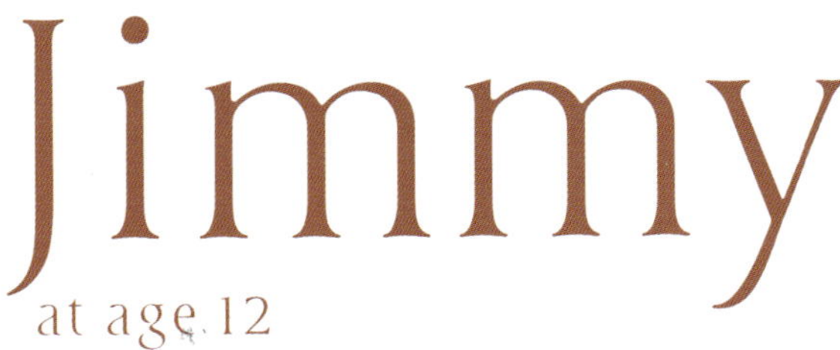

at age 12

...watching him open up.

My son Jimmy is very artistic and spontaneous. He's independent and strong-minded. He thinks a lot, and he can learn.

Every day is an experience with Jimmy — watching him open up. It's up to my husband and me, and the family, to teach him how to be a strong, independent young man, even with autism. It's another challenge for him to become stronger.

When you love somebody you do all you can for them. It's instinctive. You love your son, and you find out everything you can to help him grow. I see how our strength has helped him grow, and he's blossomed.

~Patricia, Jimmy's mother

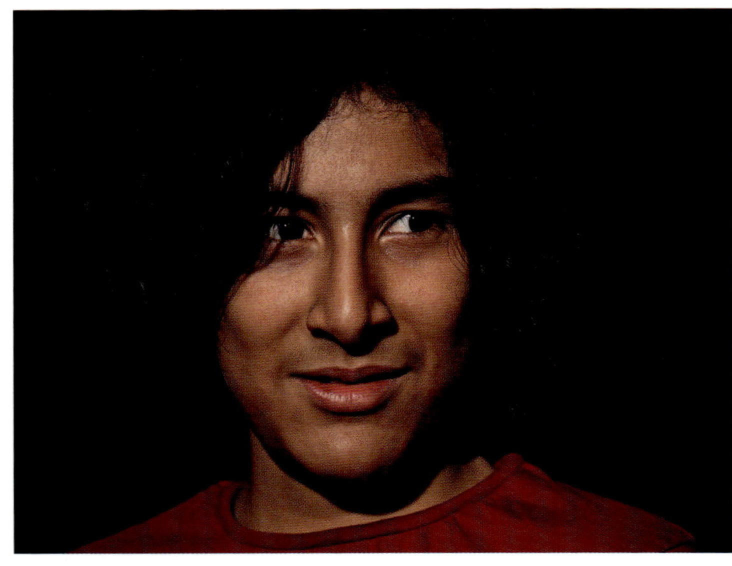

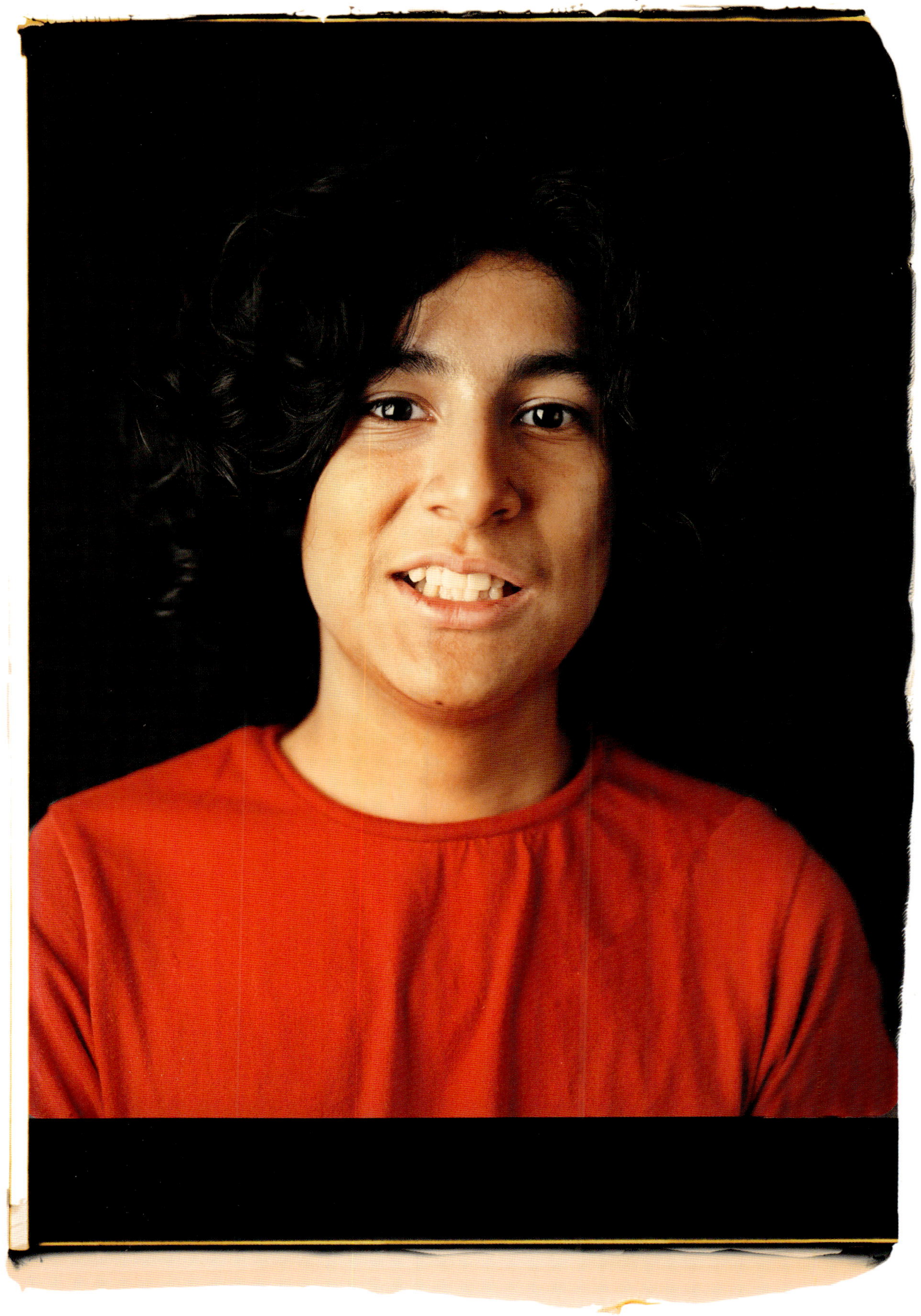

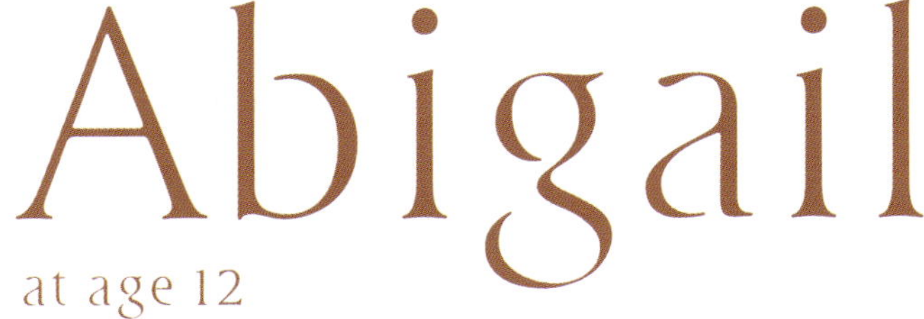

Abigail

...singing is her thing.

Abigail is a wonderful person. She's very loving, very caring and very smart. It's not about focusing on Abigail's disabilities, but focusing on the things that she's able to accomplish.

Abigail likes to sing a lot — singing is her thing. She likes music and is in a children's choir at school. When she sings, she pours out her heart, and really feels it.

She's very happy when her mom and I are together just having a good time.... every time we're together she puts her arms up and hugs the two of us.

~Adrian, Abigail's father

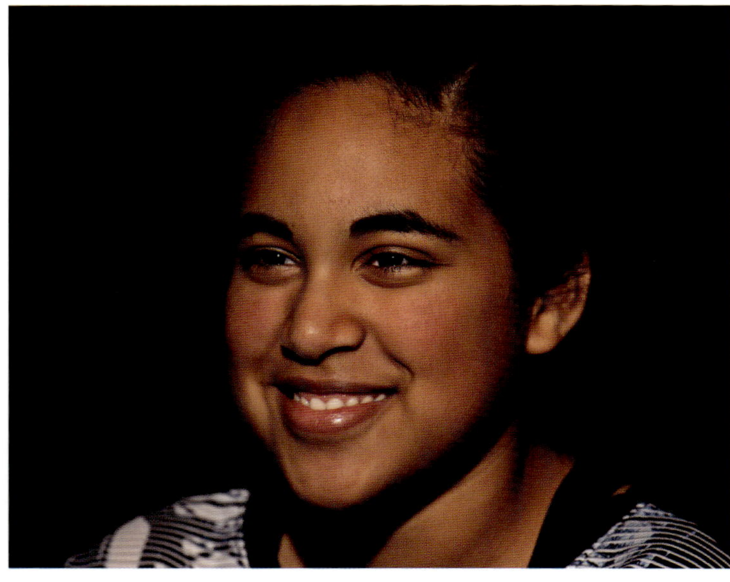

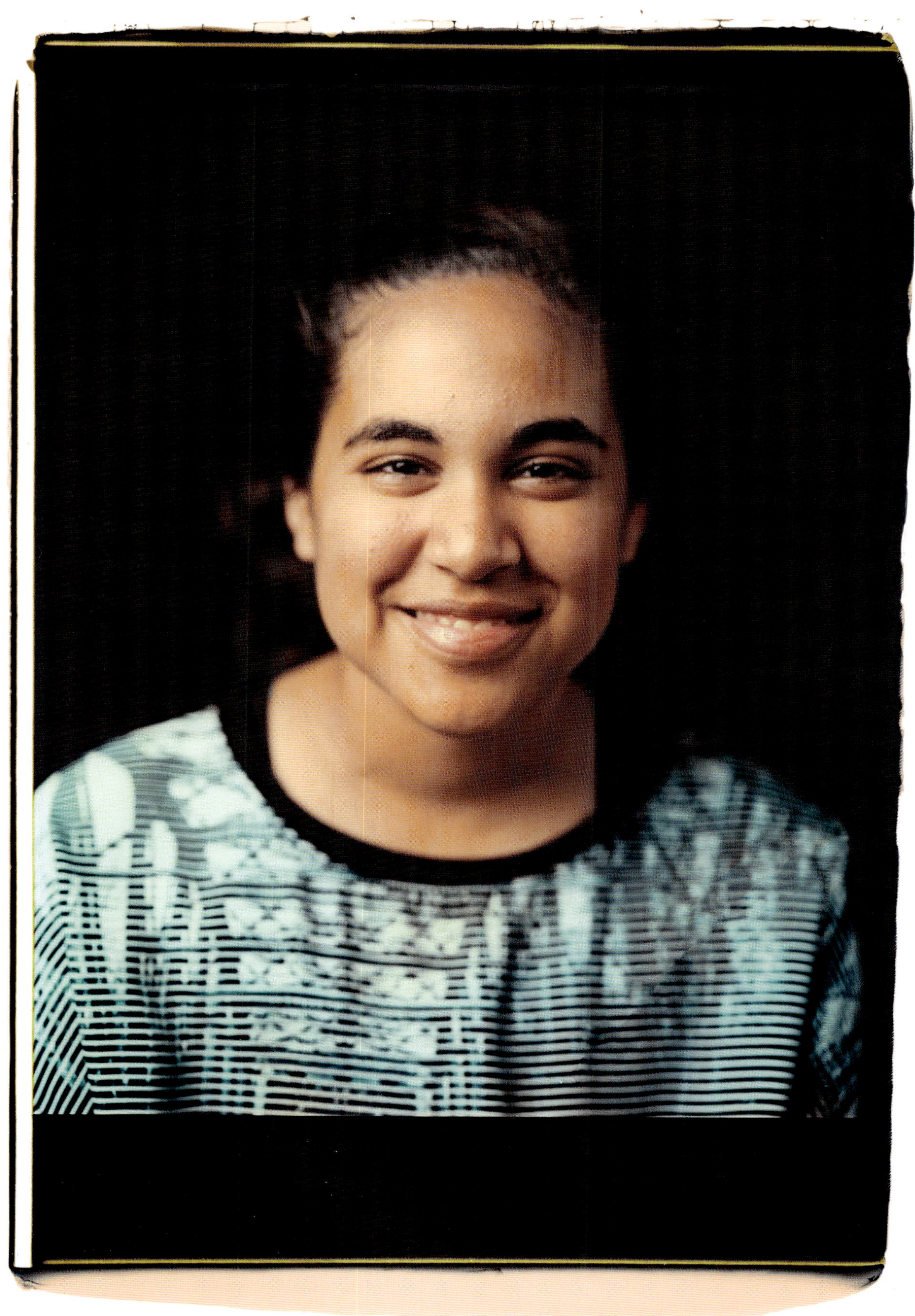

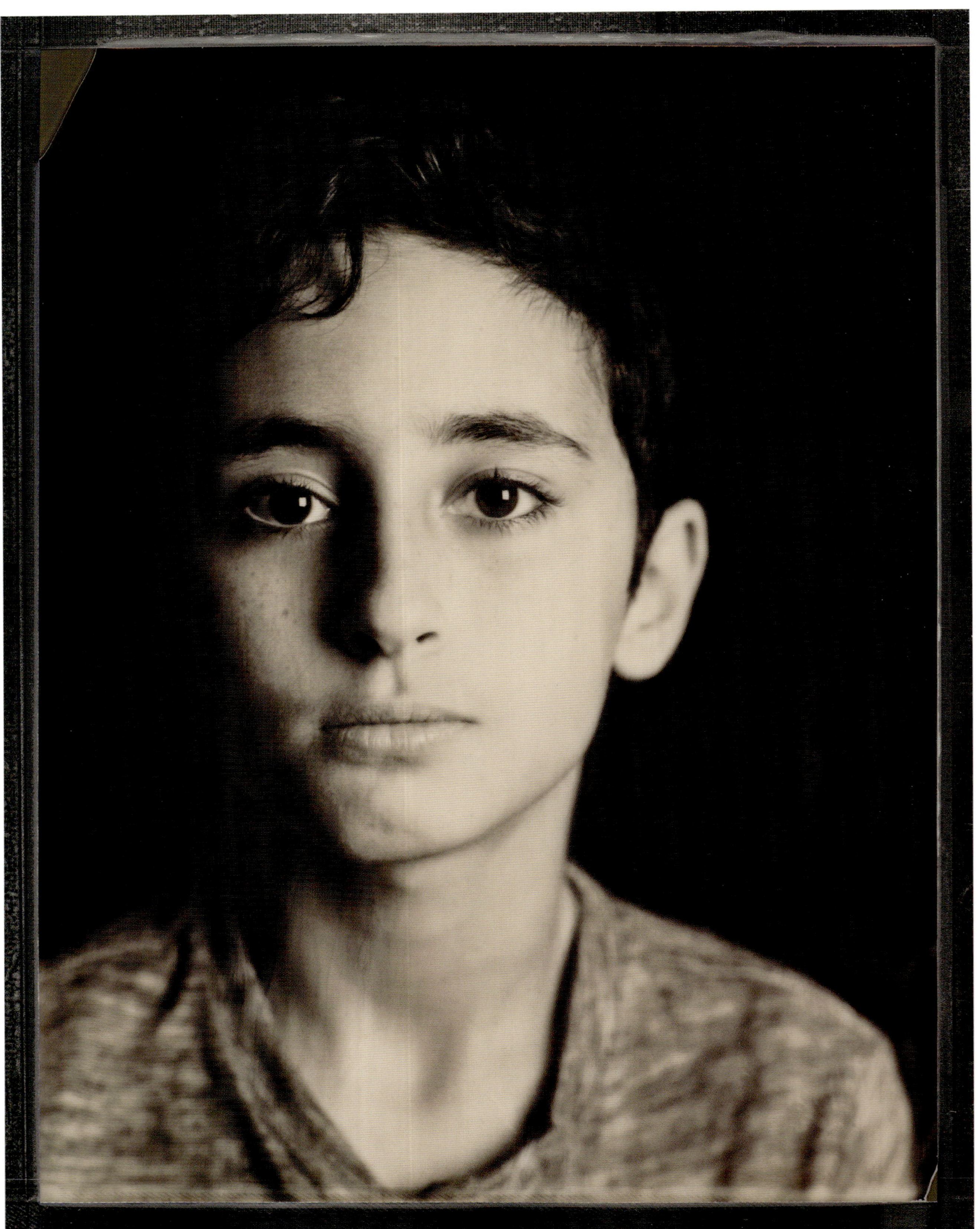

Michael

at age 12

It takes a village...

It's not the things Michael doesn't have, it's the things that he does have. He's got character. He's a comedian. He can create something from nothing. If you put him in the right situation, and the right environment, Michael can be extremely productive.

One of my plans for the future is to create a vocational training space for him, and for others. You've heard the expression, 'It takes a village to raise a child'. My wife and I are members of the village, you're a member, and everybody should be. It takes a village to raise a child with autism.

~Vartan, Michael's father

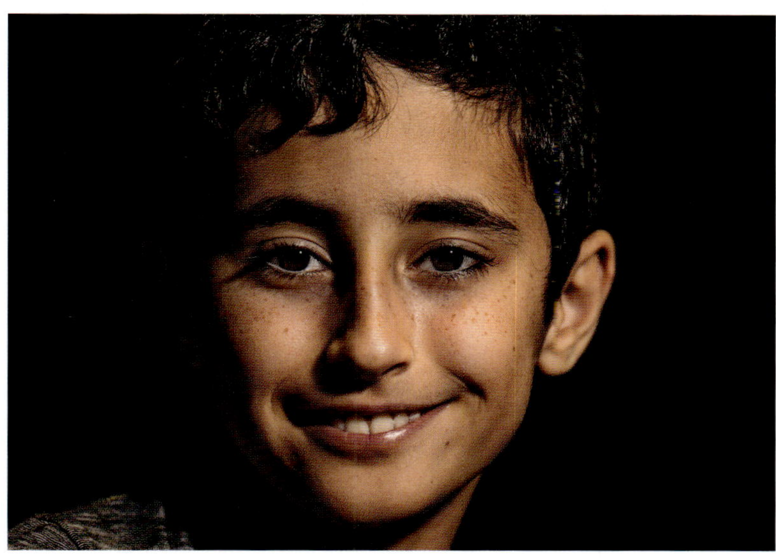

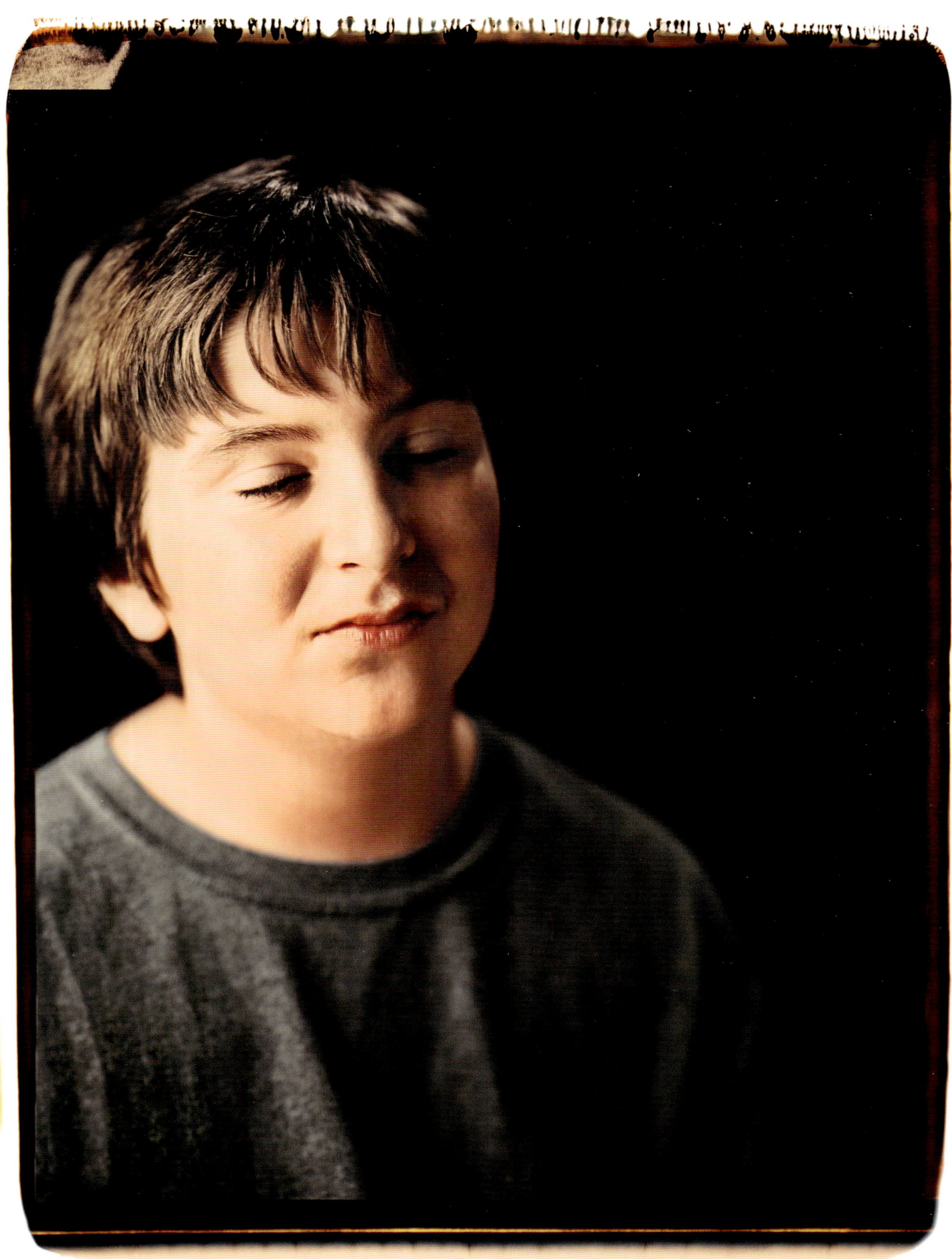

Henry

...one of the most beautiful things...

Henry is a valuable human being that deserves a place in our community. I want Henry to feel needed, and to feel like he's a part of his community — because he really is. Sometimes people can forget to step back and appreciate Henry, and what he brings to the table. He's funny, imaginative, sassy, fun to be around and energetic.

I want people to understand that Henry is a regular person in so many ways. The extraordinarily hard work that he has to do to be who he is, and to fit in, is amazing to me, and it's one of the most beautiful things that I've ever seen.

~Leah, Henry's mother

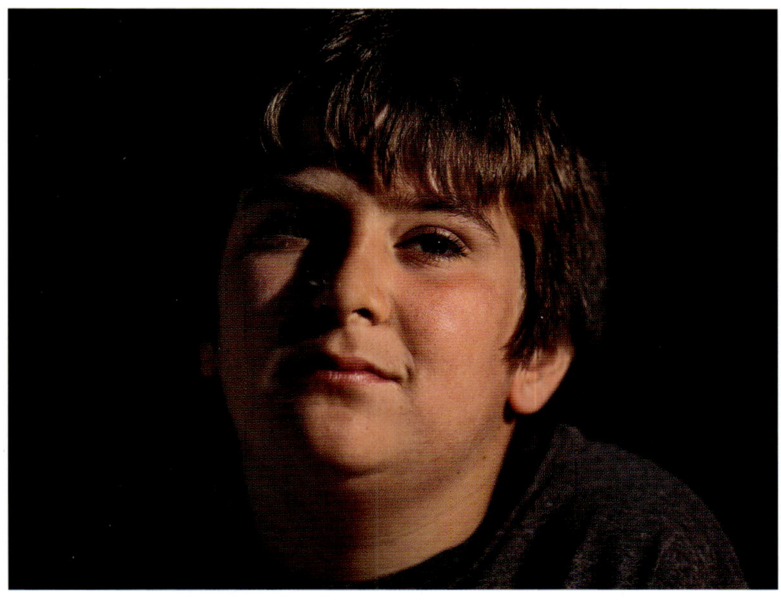

Rakim

at age 12

...at the core of Rakim...

Rakim has always been a very loving and affectionate child. He's always been very liked and we feel blessed for that. There's something about his spirit that draws people towards him.

I have a music career as did my late husband, so music is definitely a part of Rakim. When I put songs on the radio, he'll be singing along. At times when he is out of focus, we can connect together around singing. He tells me, 'Sing, sing!'. It's our special connection.

There's a certain resilience to him and an innate intelligence that's there. With continued support over the years, I hope we can really tap into what's there at the core of Rakim, and to know that there's a lot more to him than just the fact that he has autism.

~Mercedes, Rakim's mother

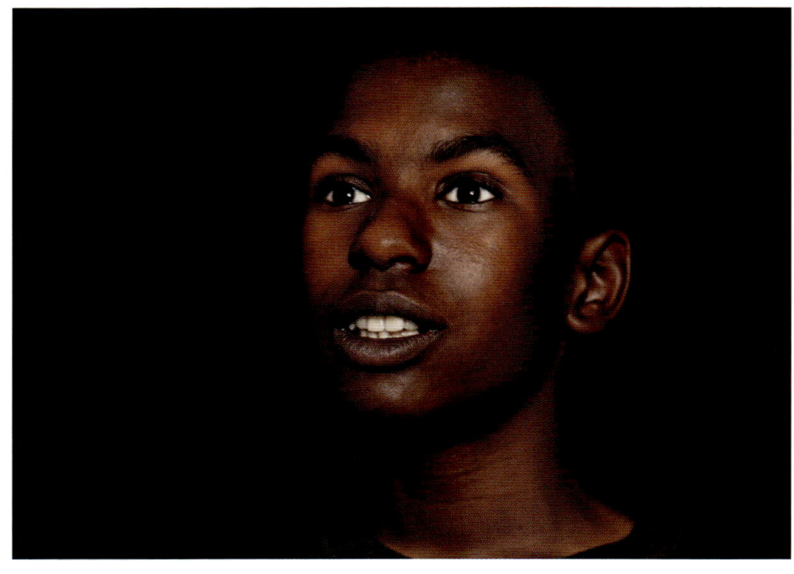

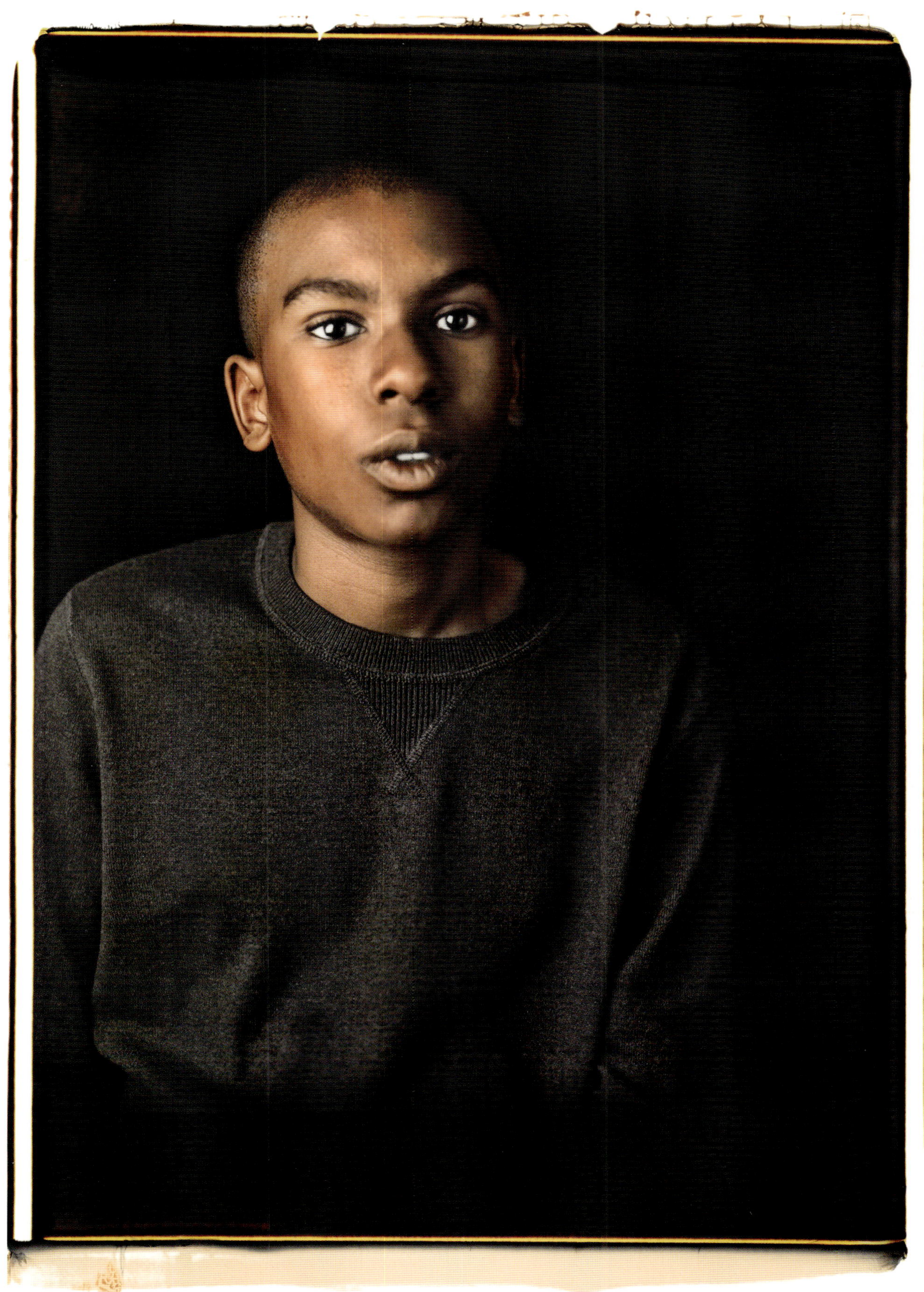

Pablo

at age 13

...fighting for a happy life.

Pabs is the strongest and most resilient person I have ever met. He's strong-willed, a fighter, and he doesn't stop fighting for a happy life. He has shown me that quitting is not an option. He makes me strive to be the best person I can be. He is a bright, shining light, even when darkness is trying to surround him. Love conquers all. And he shows us his love every single minute of every day. Our family has grown stronger with every challenge, with every obstacle that Pabs has overcome. The difficult moments have taught us to really appreciate the blessings, and seeing his big, beautiful smile is one of my family's biggest blessings.

¡Pablito ha sido un Guerrero invencible durante toda su vida; ha sido un niño con una fortaleza de acero que no se da por vencido!

~Alicia, Pablo's mother

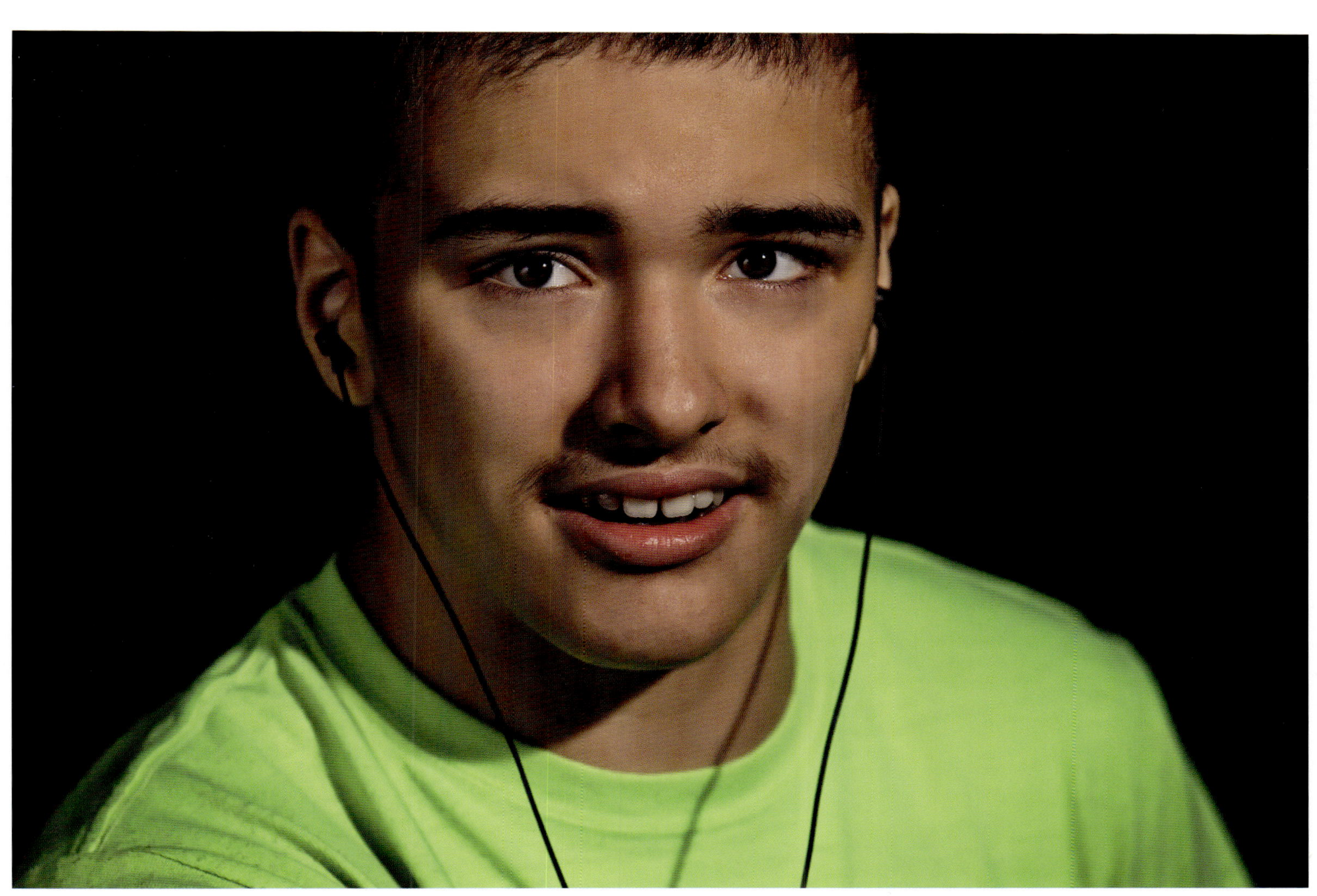

Sean & Molly

...the world through their eyes.

I want the world to know that Sean and Molly are very capable, sweet, loving, kind, affectionate, gentle human beings.

Sean and Molly have autism, and they have challenges. I like to make the analogy that they are travelers in a foreign country, and they don't speak the language, and they don't know the social cues that we all take for granted. They don't know the social graces or customs of that country.

The experiences we've shared with our children that we hold dear are the firsts, the milestones, their progress at school, their progress when they make a social connection with somebody new, when they say 'I love you'. During moments like these you see the world through their eyes.

~Jane, Sean and Molly's mother

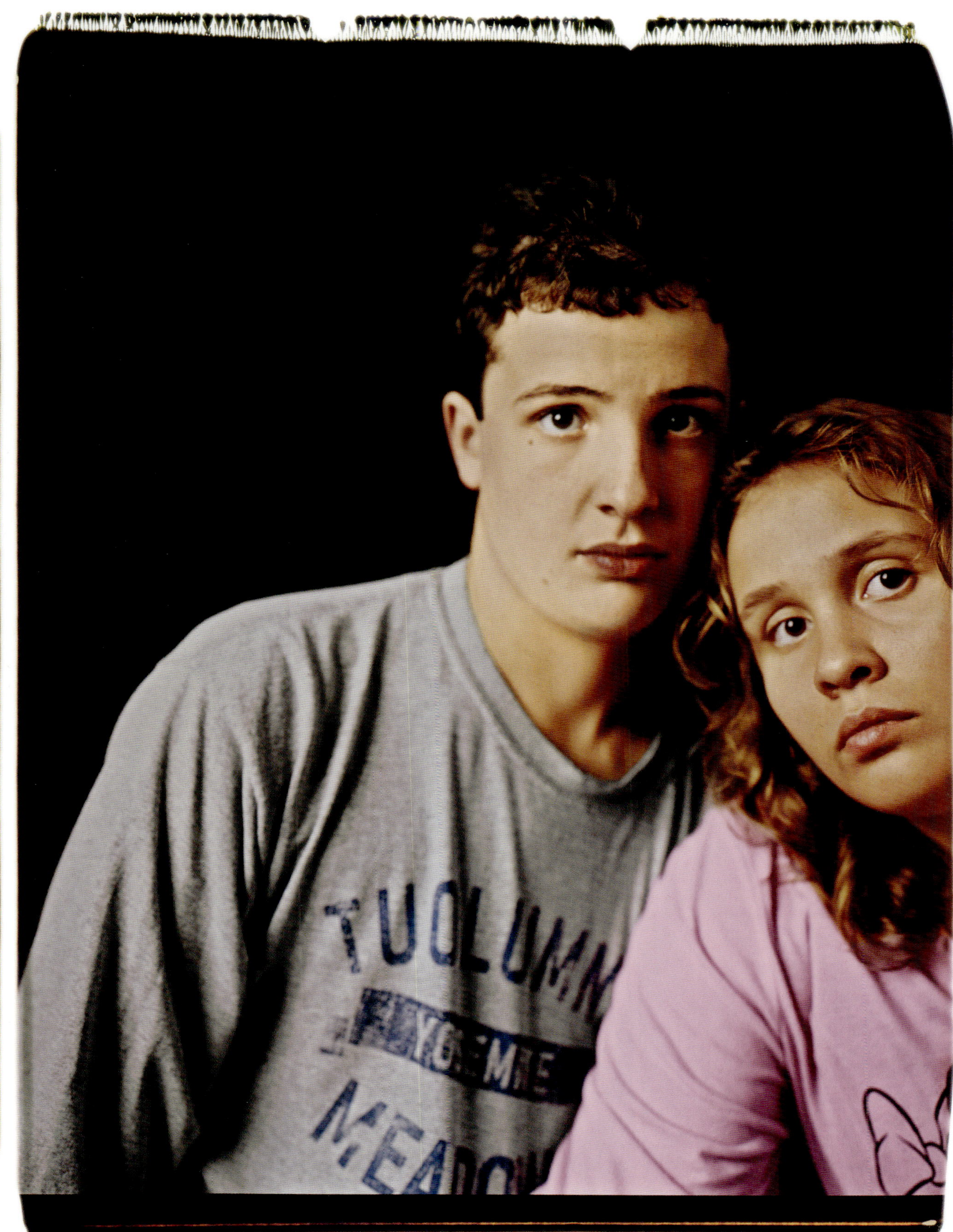
TUOLUMNE
MEADOW

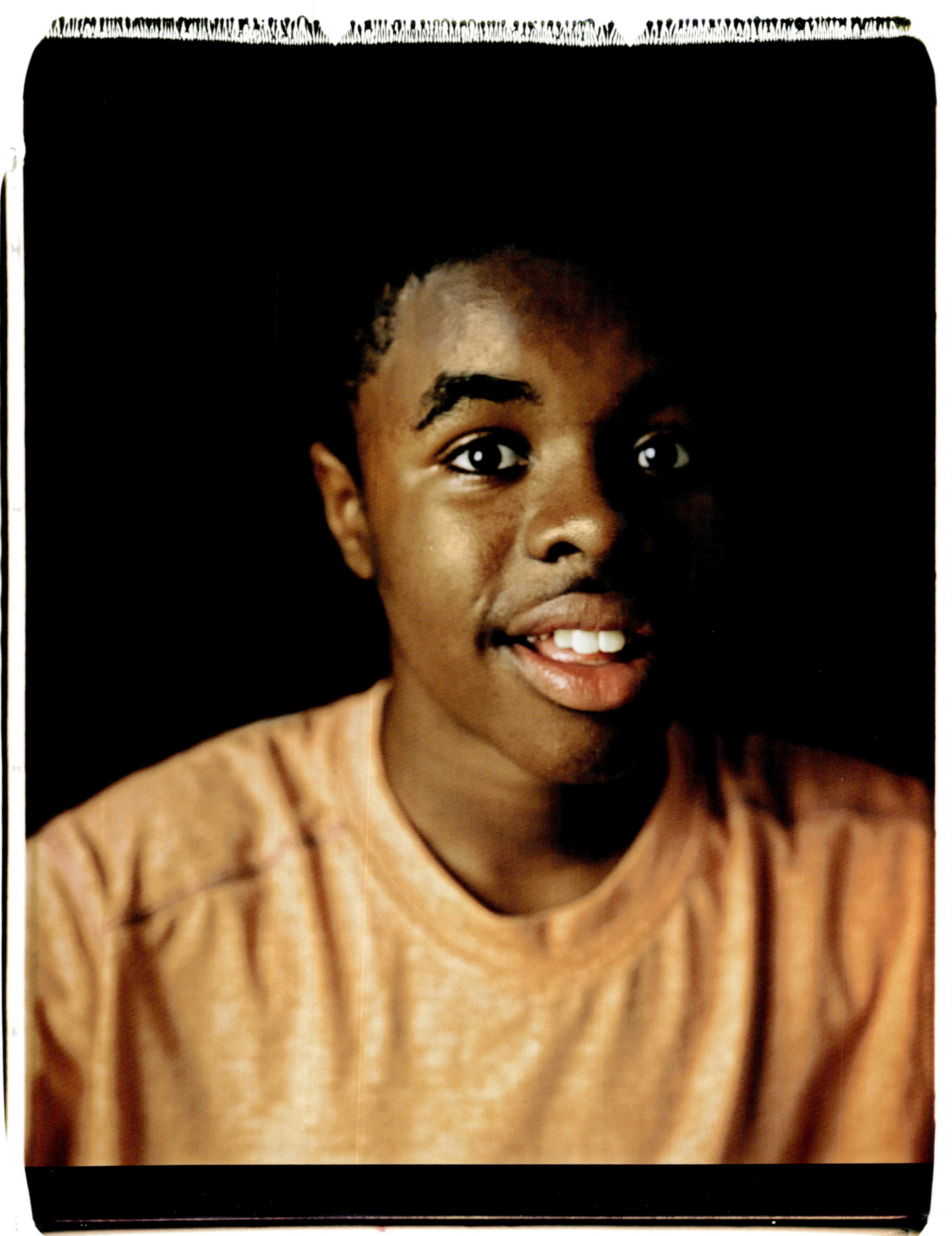

Kasten

at age 13

...not a stereotype or a label.

Kasten is a unique individual with thoughts, feelings, emotions, ideas and talent — just like the rest of us. He's an amazing human being, not a stereotype or a label. Kasten shouldn't be bullied or ostracized because he's different.

When Kasten is around us, I see confidence. He always gives me this beaming smile that just makes me melt. Whenever I walk into the room after he's been at school all day, Kasten has this special smile for mommy. Whatever my day has been like, that all goes away when I see Kasten.

~Mizpah, Kasten's mother

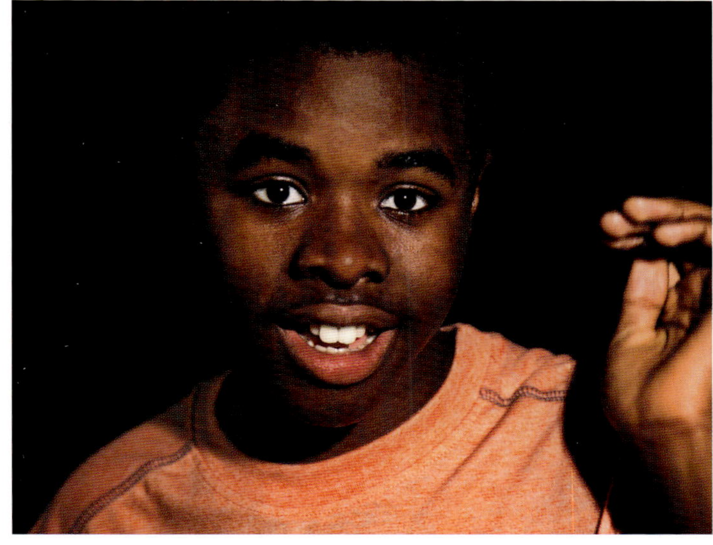 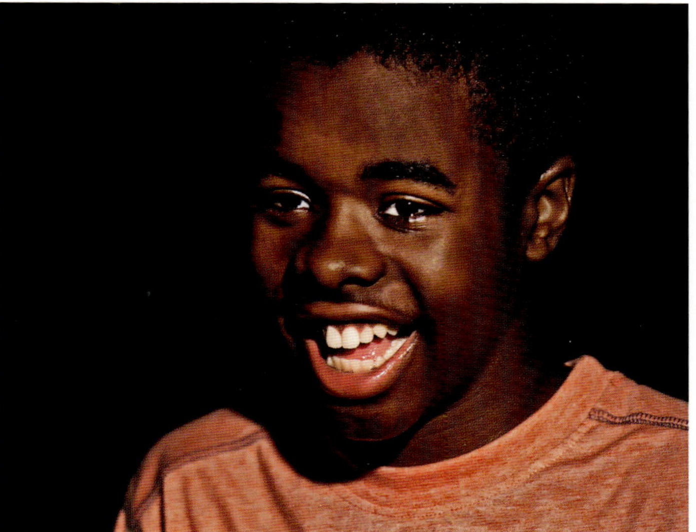

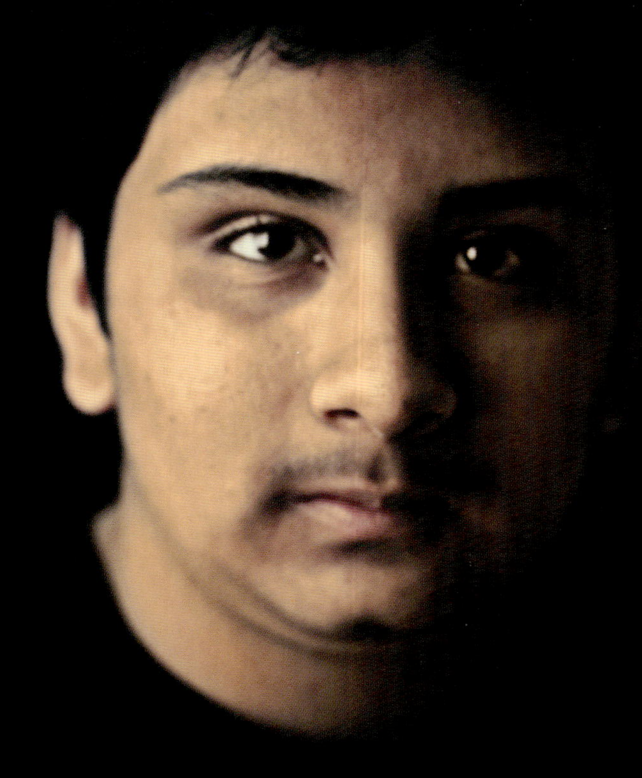
SAN FRANCI

Christopher

at age 14

...he just continues to amaze me...

I love Christopher so much. He's gone through so many different phases and he just continues to amaze me with what he's capable of doing, and how much he knows and understands.

My parents have a close relationship with Christopher. When Christopher is having a hard time, his grandpa will say, 'Let's go for a ride'. Christopher is just as happy as can be to follow his grandpa. My father knows what's going to make Christopher feel better.

I remember when Christopher tried to make my father feel better. One day, when my mom fell ill, and Christopher saw how upset my father was, he would come around and hug his grandfather. He knew something was wrong, and he was trying the best way he could to comfort him.

~Ofelia, Christopher's mother

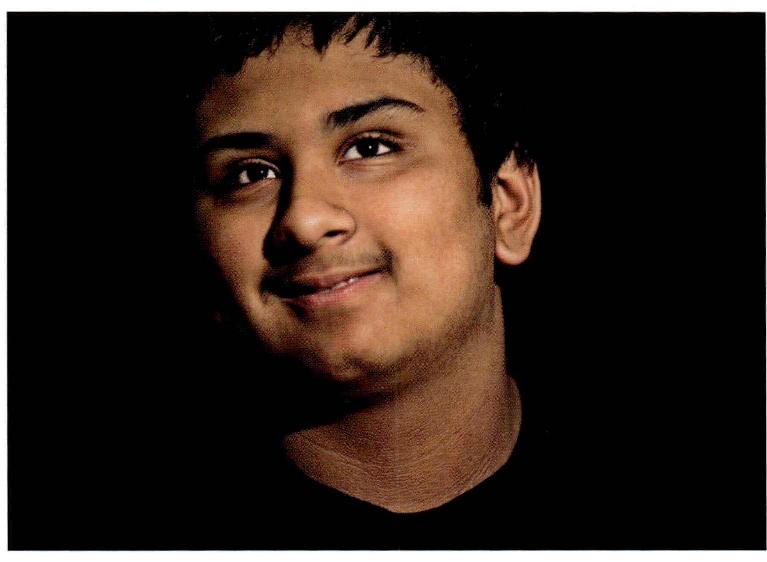

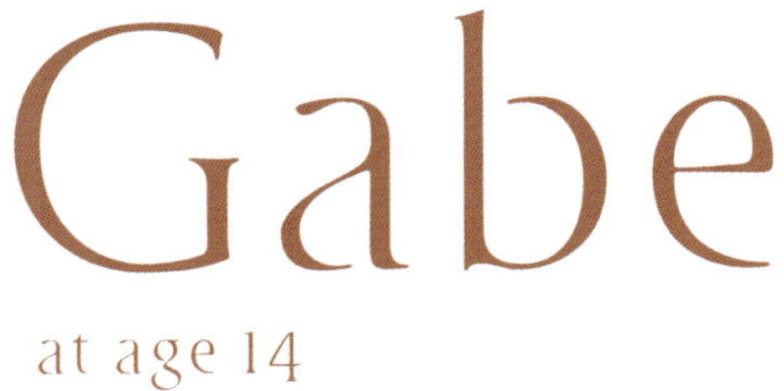

Gabe

at age 14

...to be seen as a whole person...

I really want Gabe to be seen as a whole person, not just as someone with autism. There's so much more to him and I definitely don't define him that way.

Gabe has a sense of humor and he's empathetic and flexible. He loves new people and new experiences. He's extremely social, up for a good time — all the time — a real people person. These are strengths that some people don't typically associate with individuals with autism. I want the world to see him as more like them, rather than different from them. And I want him to have access and exposure to all the things that make any life meaningful.

~Jesse, Gabe's mother

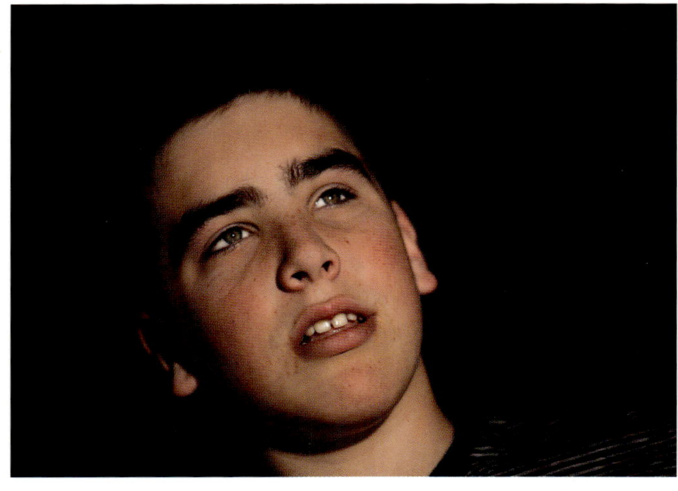

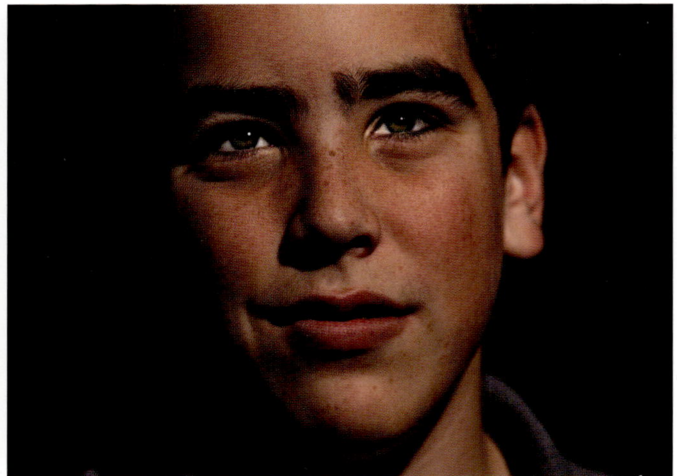

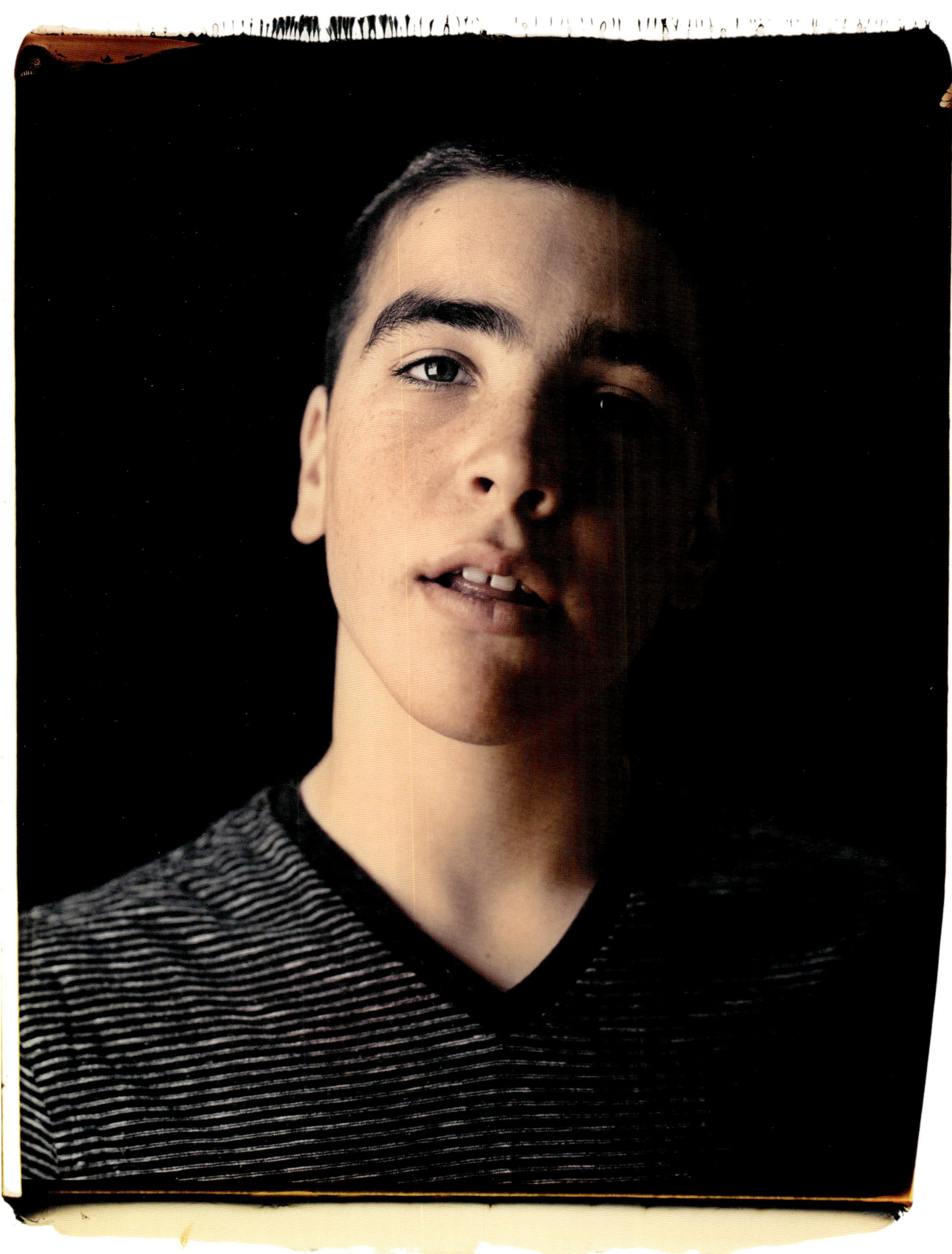

Nicholas

at age 14

...Nicholas called me mom.

I remember the first time Nicholas called me mom. That was probably the most special day in my life. He was about 10 and he just came up to me and said, 'Mom.' I couldn't even answer him because I was in tears.

Nicholas and his brother are 11 months apart. They're just typical brothers, who do what boys do. His brother told me that he wanted to be a millionaire by the time he was 23. I asked him why, and he said, 'Because I have to take care of Nick.'

~Gina, Nicholas's mother

...Nick is going to be okay.

Nicholas, like any other kid, is complex. He's not just a kid with autism. Nick is a person with a lot of emotions, challenges, accomplishments, joys and disappointments — his experiences are as rich and varied as all of ours.

Nick loves the beach. I have a wonderful memory of him in the water. There was a wave coming and he just opened his arms and let the wave hit him and it was just one of the most amazing things I ever saw. For me, seeing that made me feel like Nick is going to be okay.

~Gary, Nicholas's father

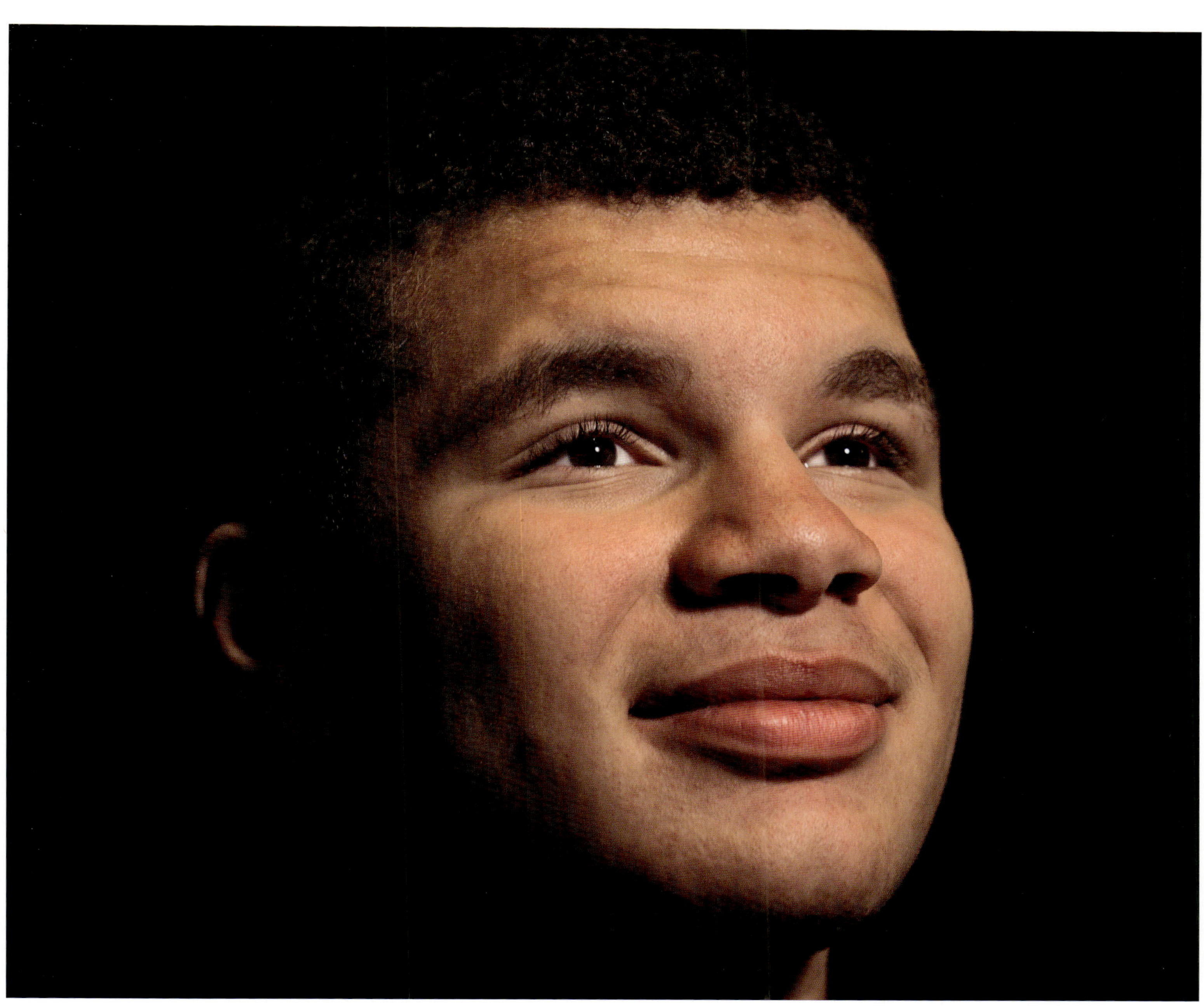

Britney & Adrian

siblings, at ages 15 and 13

...a good brother and sister.

When Britney had a starring role in Peter Pan at school, I was so happy and amazed that she could do that. She had very high self–esteem, and felt the praise from the people around her.

Adrian is a very happy child and since he was little he's just the kind of person you'd like to have as a friend. Britney takes care of Adrian — she's always looking out for him. Whenever Adrian sees Britney feeling sad or mad, or crying, he tells her, 'Britney, it's okay.'

~Jose, Britney's and Adrian's father

Britney and Adrian are very attached to each other. They spend time together at school, and they share some of the same feelings. It makes me happy that they respect each other. They help each other. They're a good brother and sister.

~Noraelsa, Britney's and Adrian's mother

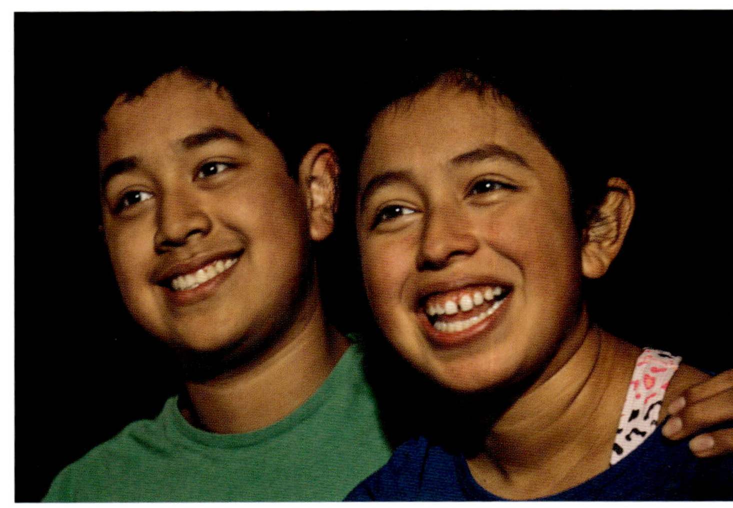

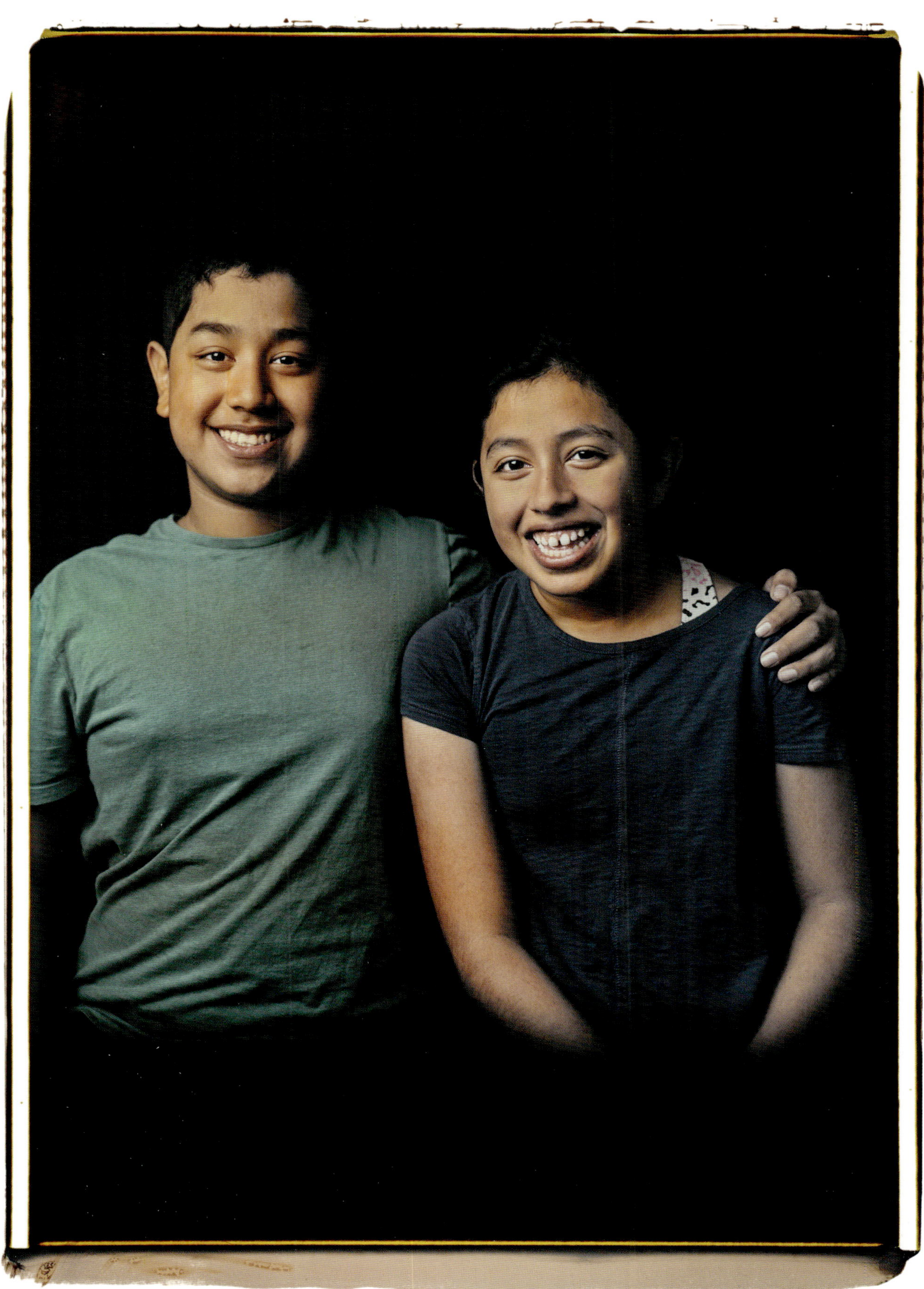

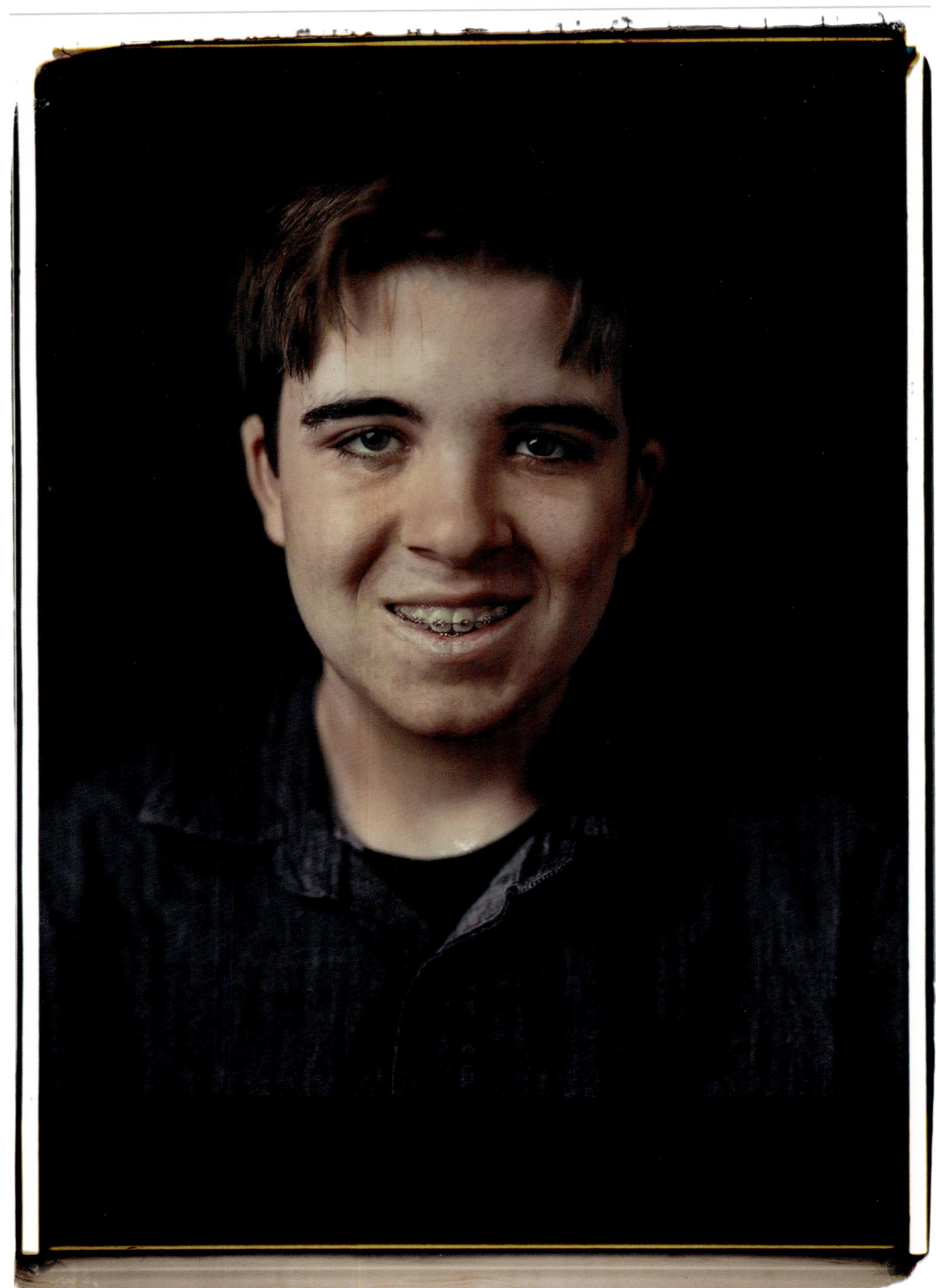

Thaddeus

at age 15

...that proud look on his face...

I want people to know Thaddeus has so many different layers. When he expresses himself through art, Thaddeus really starts shining. He sang on stage at the Sonoma Film Festival. It was amazing, and I cried. It's that proud look on his face and in his eyes. I can be proud of him all day long, but when he's proud of himself, that's it. That's the deal.

Thaddeus has challenges, like in math and in social situations, but he's a really hard worker. One day he went surfing, and he wiped out. He interpreted that as failure. A surfer on the beach encouraged him, 'Wipeouts are the best. You go out, you wipe out, and you come back.' And so we started talking about wipeouts in a metaphoric way, in relation to practicing, and getting good at something. It was a life-changing event, all of a sudden he was like, 'Yeah, I can practice it'.

~Kristin, Thaddeus's mother

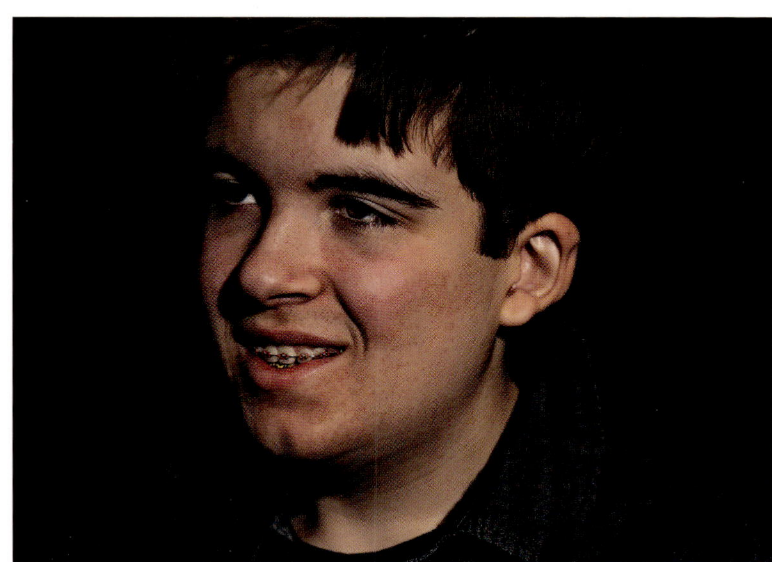

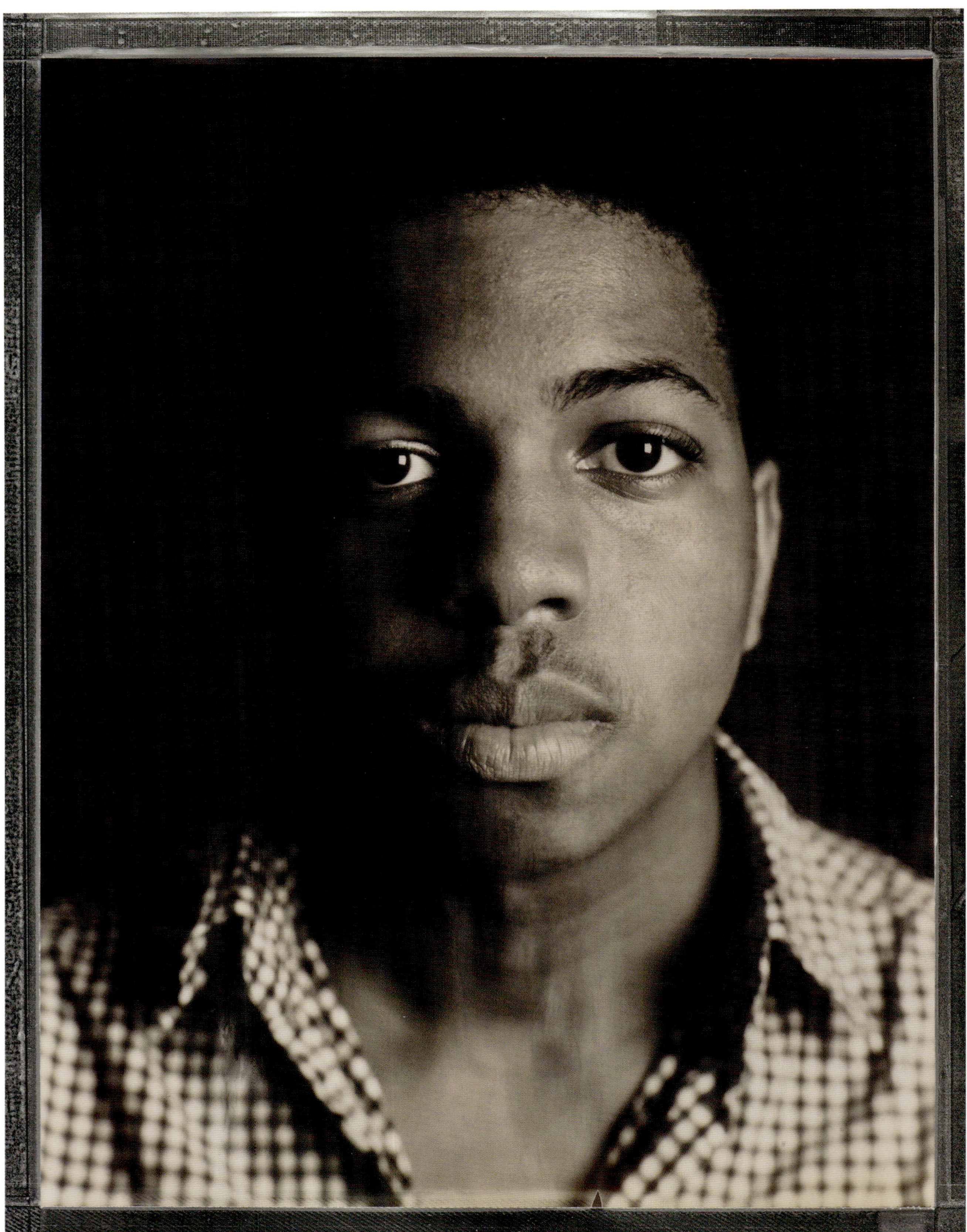

Chester

at age 15

He can do it.

Chester is able to see the good in everybody. He's my master teacher for kindness, graciousness, gratitude and generosity. He really has that embedded in him as a human being and that has nothing to do with a diagnosis. He makes me really proud. When he walks through the world, he does it with such dignity. I don't want him to be seen as a diagnosis, as a gender, as a race. I want Chester to be seen as a whole human being, fully realized, authentic.

My hope for Chester is that he reaches his dreams, and that he doesn't allow anything to stop him from being the person he knows he is inside. He can do it.

~Kimberly, Chester's mother

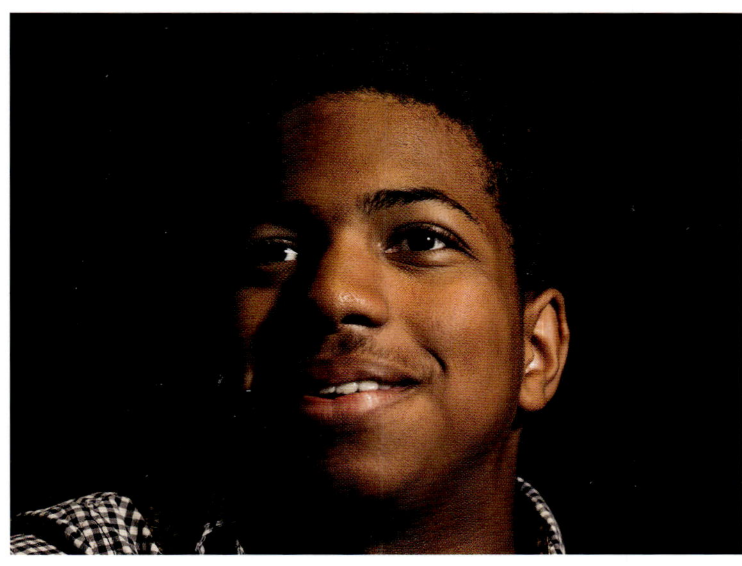

Cullen

...a very gratifying feeling.

I want to show people that having autism isn't causing me to fall back. I'm keeping pace despite it, with it and in some cases being helped along because of it.

I keep working, and trying to improve. I'd say my biggest strength would be math. I want to study math in college. When I was younger my preference was to learn by myself. Now, in my school's STEM program, working with my teammates is very challenging, but it's very fulfilling to know that you are able to come together with people, and to do something cooperatively. It is a very gratifying feeling.

~Cullen, in his own words

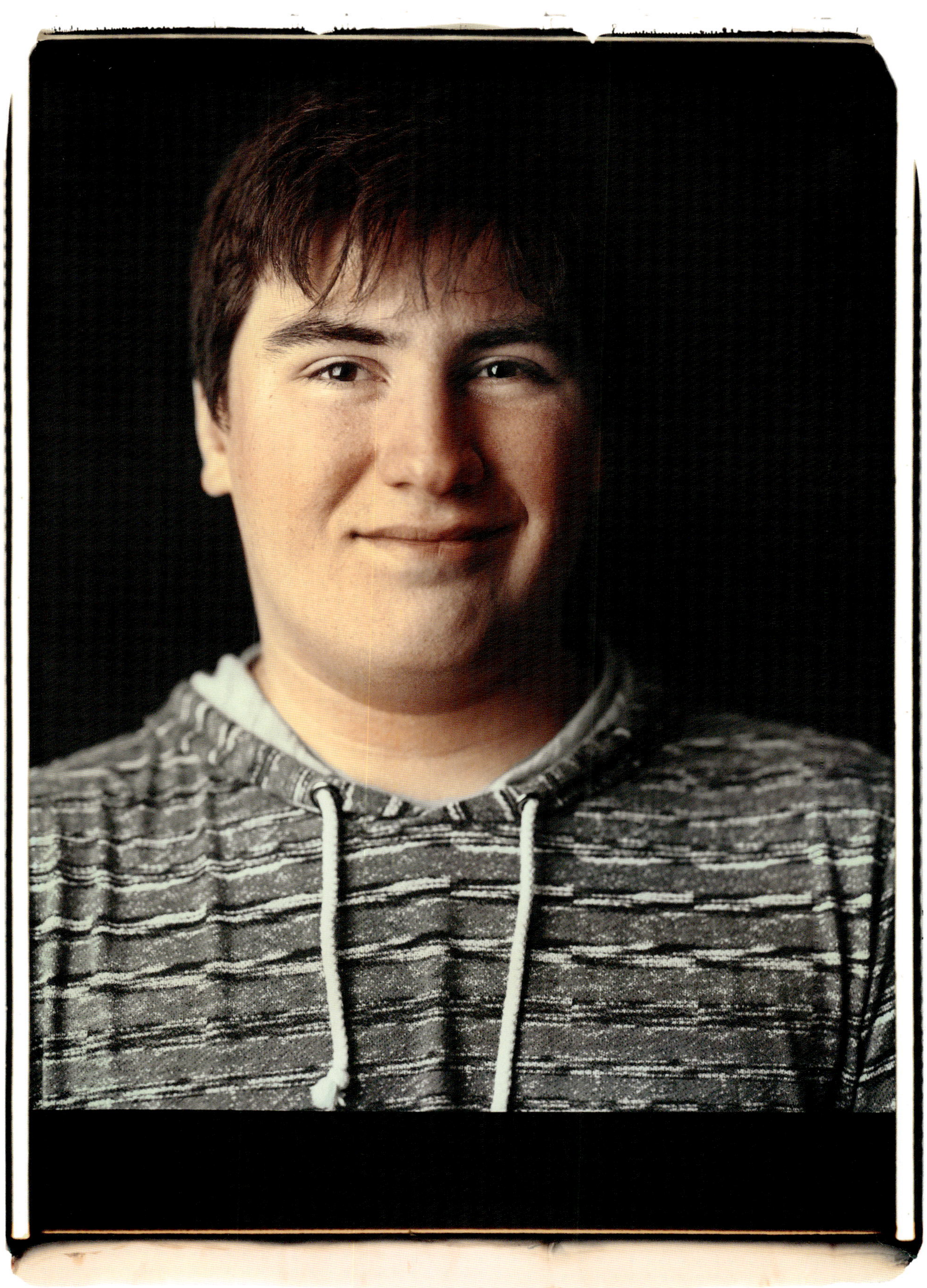

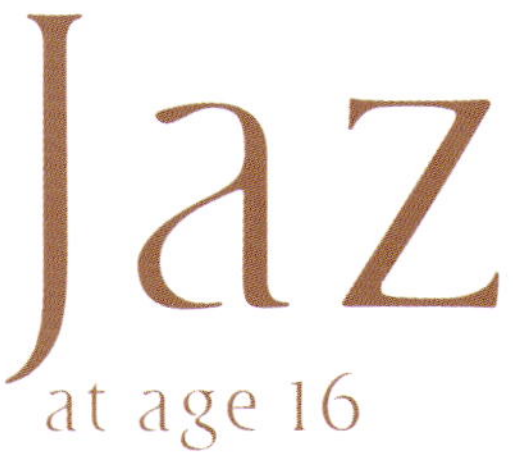

Jaz
at age 16

I feel accepted.

Jaz likes to take bike rides in our community. I asked him, 'What is it about the bike rides that you gotta get on your bike every day and gotta ride?' And then he said, 'You know what mom, I love this community. I feel accepted. I love riding my bike on Ventura Boulevard and looking in the shops, and I know everyone in some of the stores and they know me.'

That feeling of acceptance in a community, how it strengthened him in his heart, and in his abilities to perform in school and life, and to excel — that's what it's about.

~Kelly, Jaz's mother

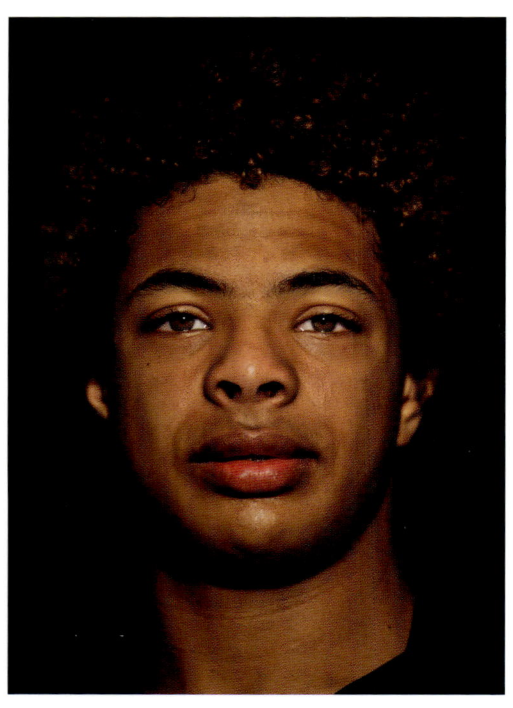

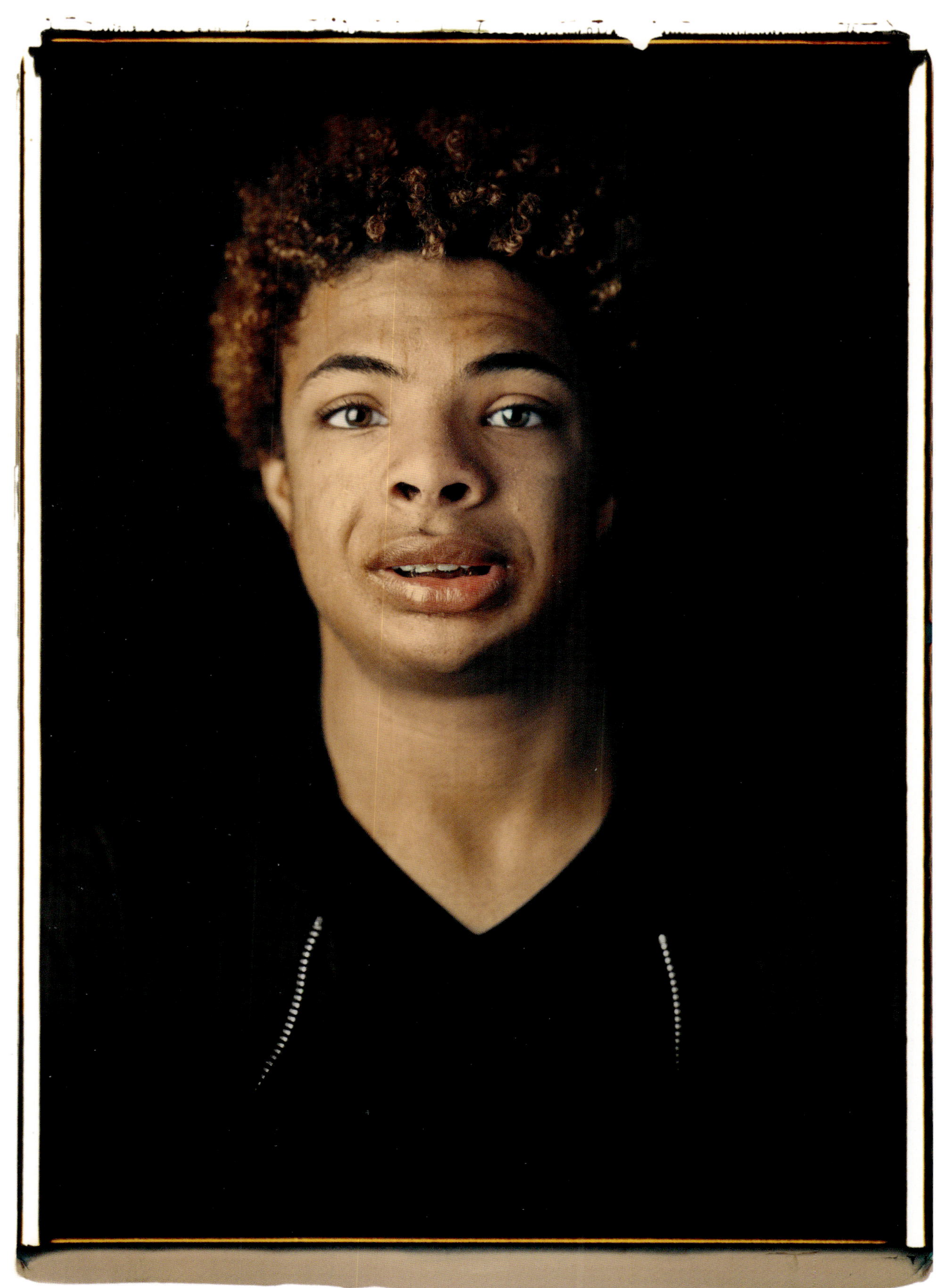

Ben

at age 17

I'm going to college.

It hasn't always been easy for me. It wasn't until I was 13 or 14 that I realized I had strengths in computers and math. I like those two things, they kinda go hand-in-hand. My school's robotics team played a big part of furthering my interests. I was the programmer on my school's team, which was kinda fun. It was definitely a lot of teamwork. I was also called, 'Mr. IT'. If anyone had a problem with their computer they would call me.

I like to play the guitar and bass. About a year ago, I decided to try and learn the bass, which is more rhythmic.

I'm going to college. I'd like to find some kind of job in the software engineering field.

~Ben, in his own words

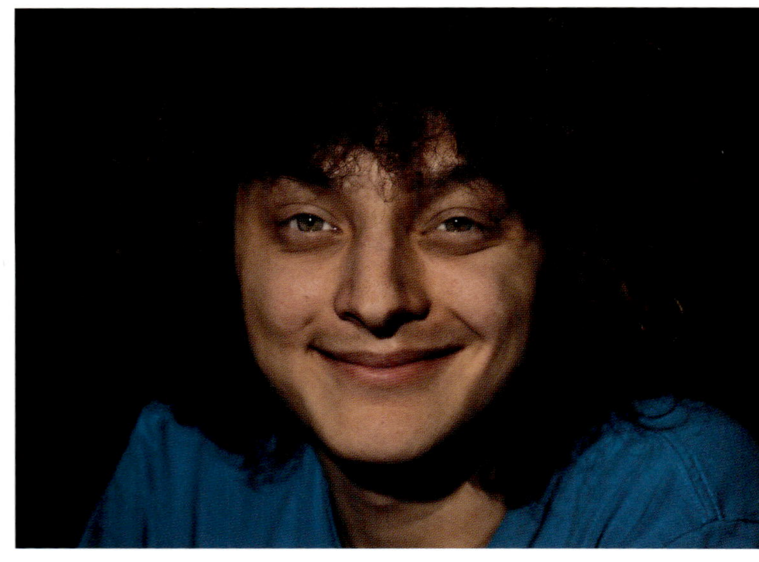

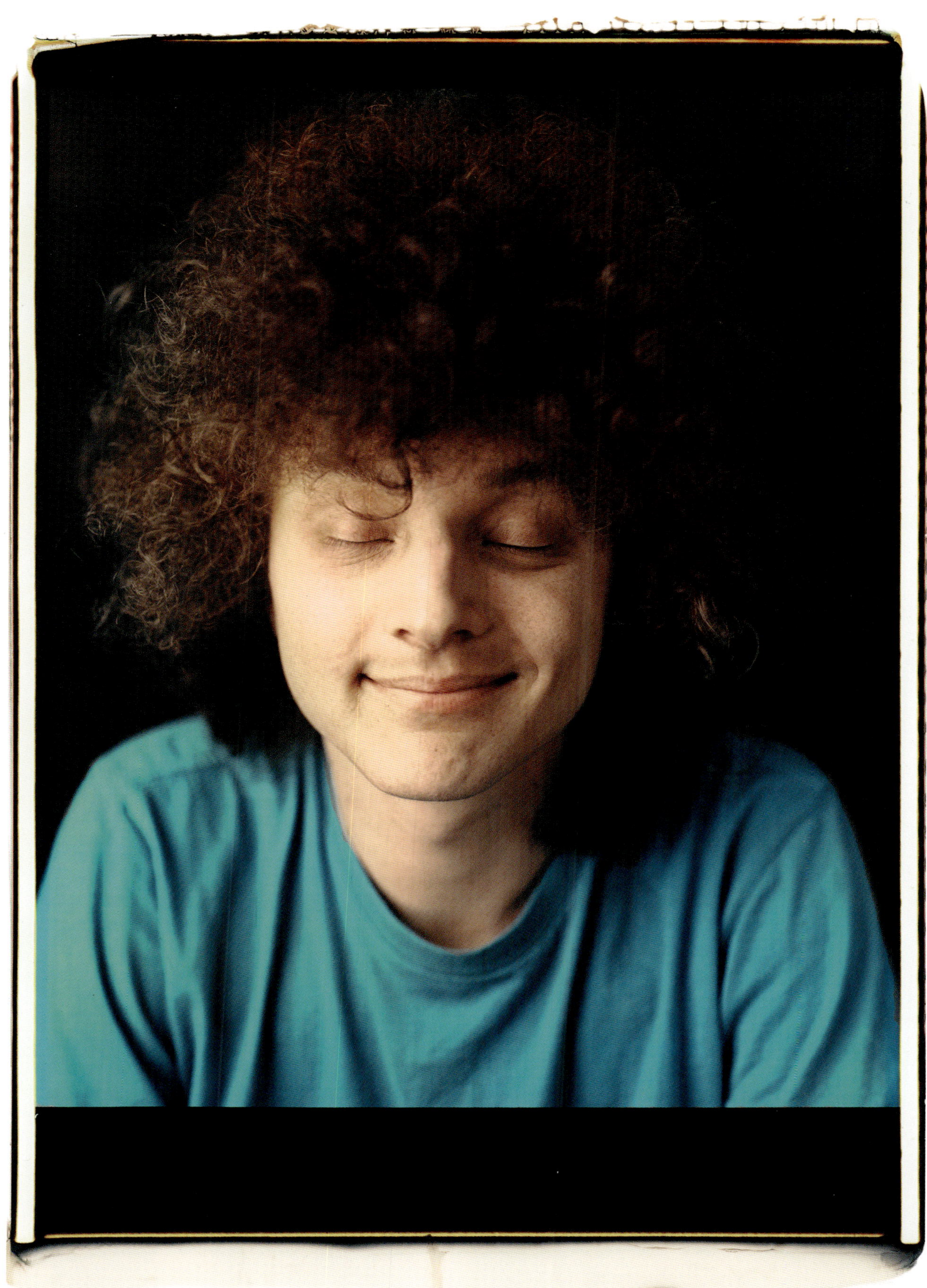

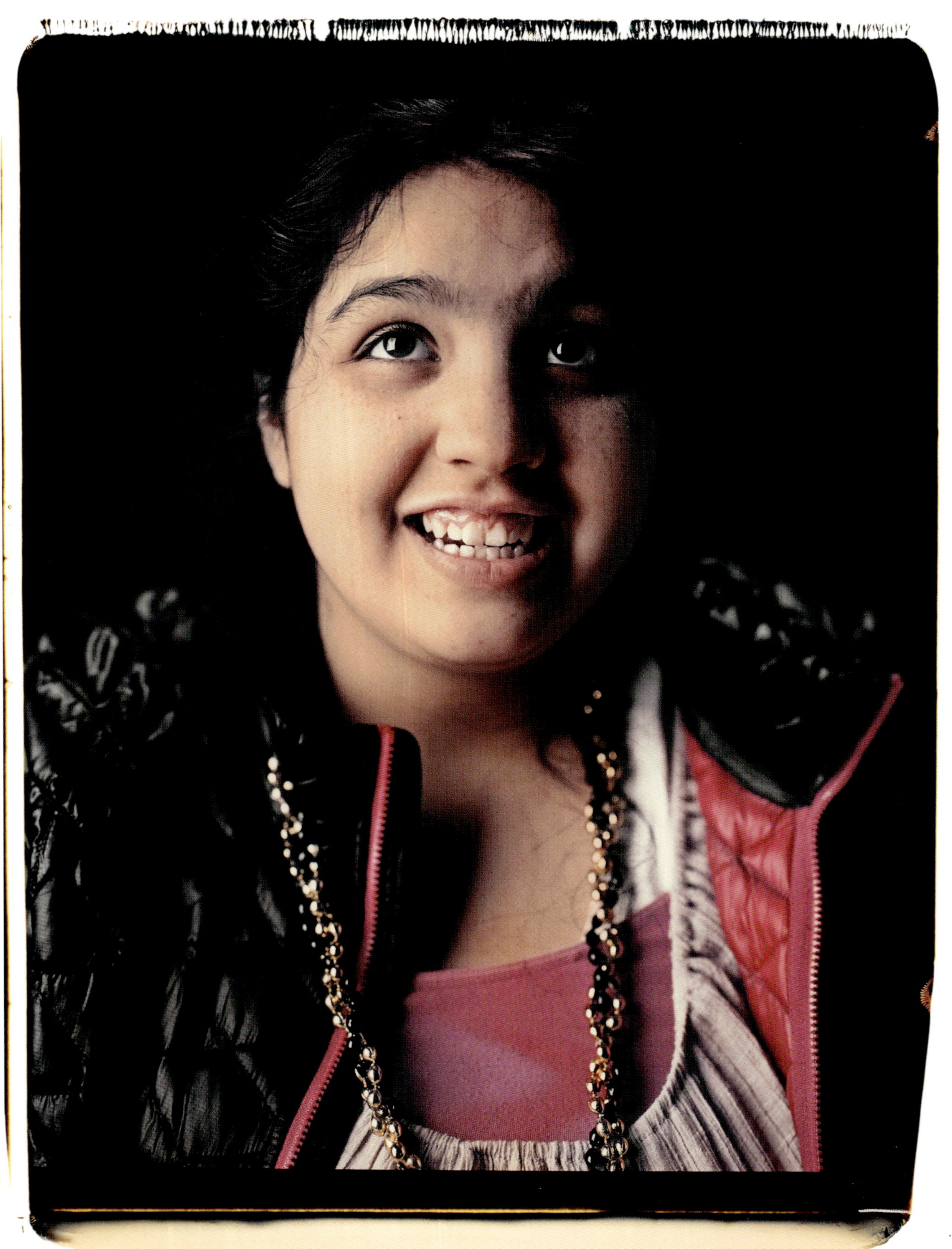

Savanna

Savanna blossoms...

Sometimes children with autism have a hard time making friendships because they don't know how to socialize. Savanna now has a friend at school. When I saw Savanna holding her friend's hand in a school picture it was so endearing to me.

Savanna has a sister who is 18 months older. They have developed a beautiful relationship over the past 3 years. They wash the dogs together — that's their thing right now.

Savanna blossoms when she's out in the community. She loves riding the bus and working at her job. I think Savanna feels important, and it's giving her more confidence.

~Teresa, Savanna's mother

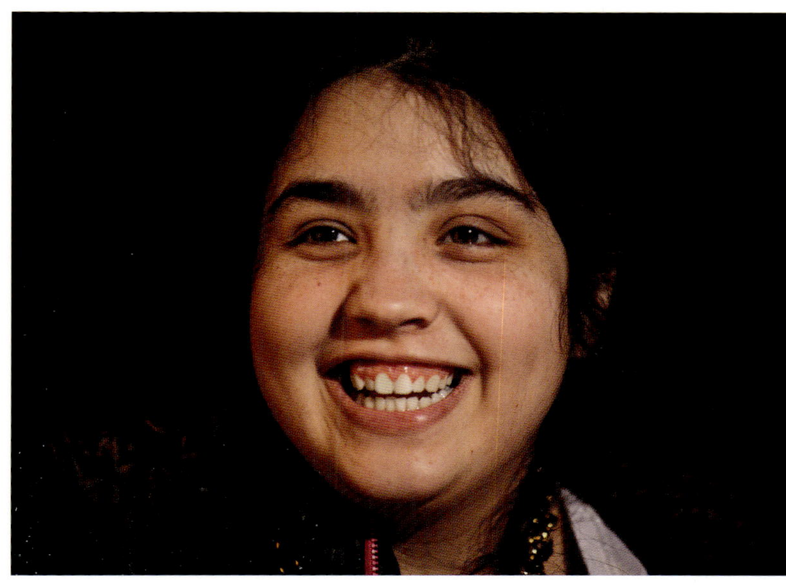

Tali
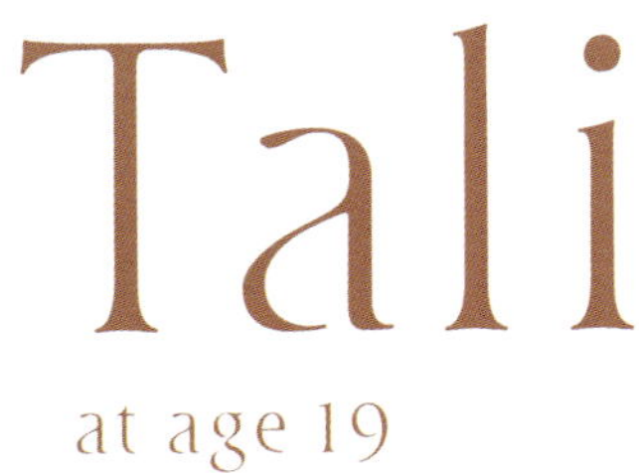
at age 19

...the heart of our family...

Our daughter Tali, who has severe disabilities, is the heart of our family, and everyone has grown. Tali brings soul and heart, and learning to just love unconditionally.

My husband and I attended her prom. I was so proud to be one of the mom's who got their daughter ready for prom. To pick out a dress, put on a little makeup, and watch her so excited — it was a wonderful feeling for my husband and me. Now both of our daughters have been to proms.

The world does see Tali. Most people look past the disability because there's a sense of pureness with her. She is such a loving, warm person. She's fun and makes you feel good about you.

~Allison, Tali's mother

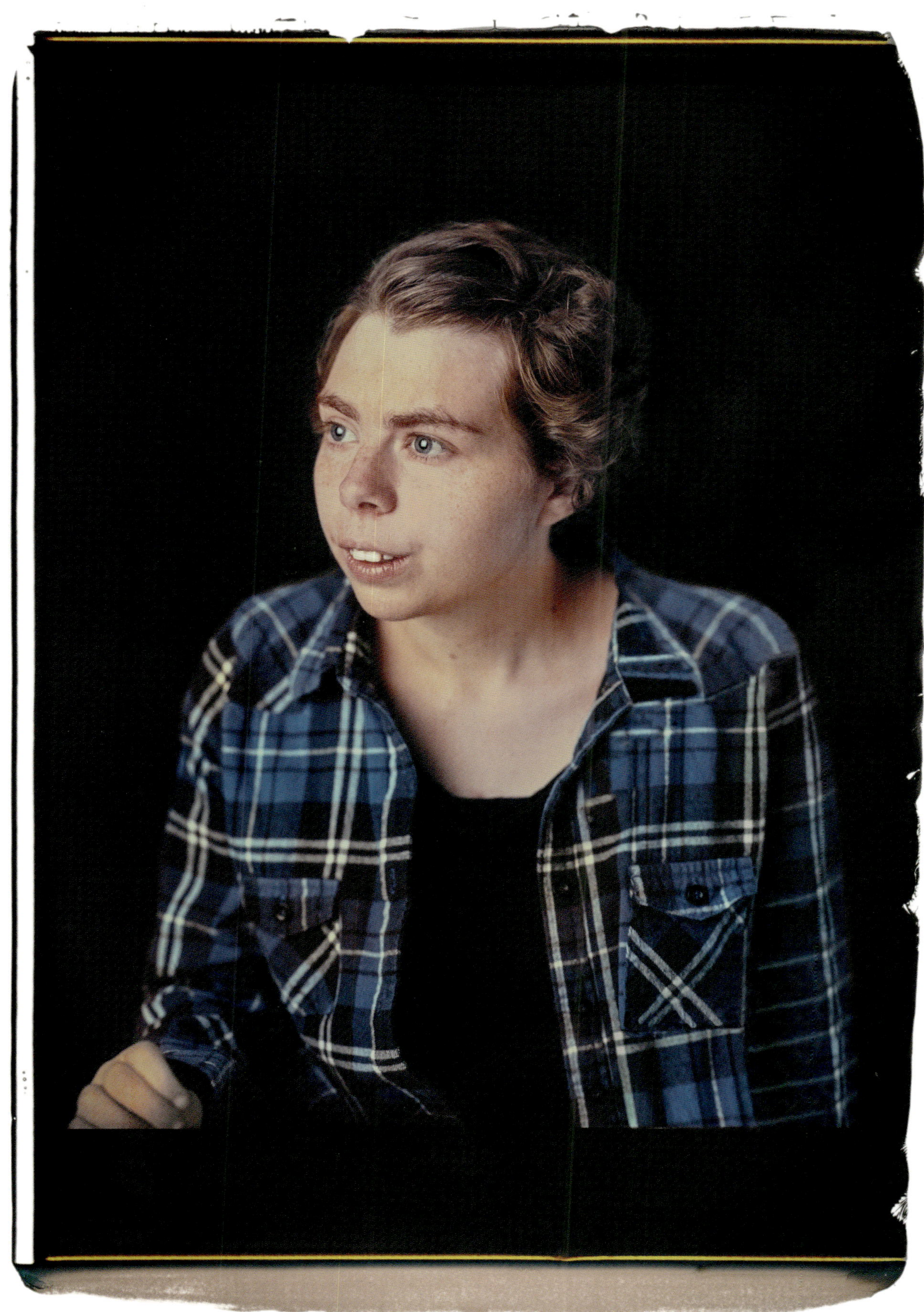

Alex

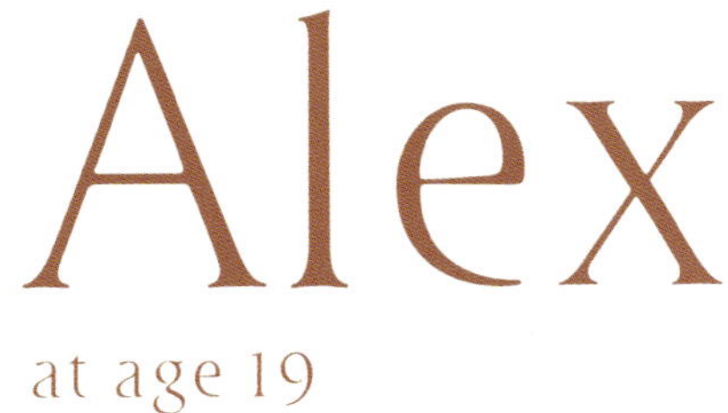

at age 19

...a purity of emotion...

Alex is an integral part of our family, and our lives are richer because of him. He has a purity of emotion that is not seen in other people. Alex is happy, he's always laughing and enjoying things. We can't imagine life without him. It's the closeness of our family relationship that gives us strength.

Alex's two sisters and his brother adore him and they've gone through a lot together. They've internalized a duty to be supportive of Alex, and have even pursued helping professions.

Alex is capable of loving. I want people to look at Alex and know that he has a contribution to make.

~Mimi, Alex's mother

I want people to be more aware of autism, and to be understanding. We can all learn something from Alex.

~Lan, Alex's father

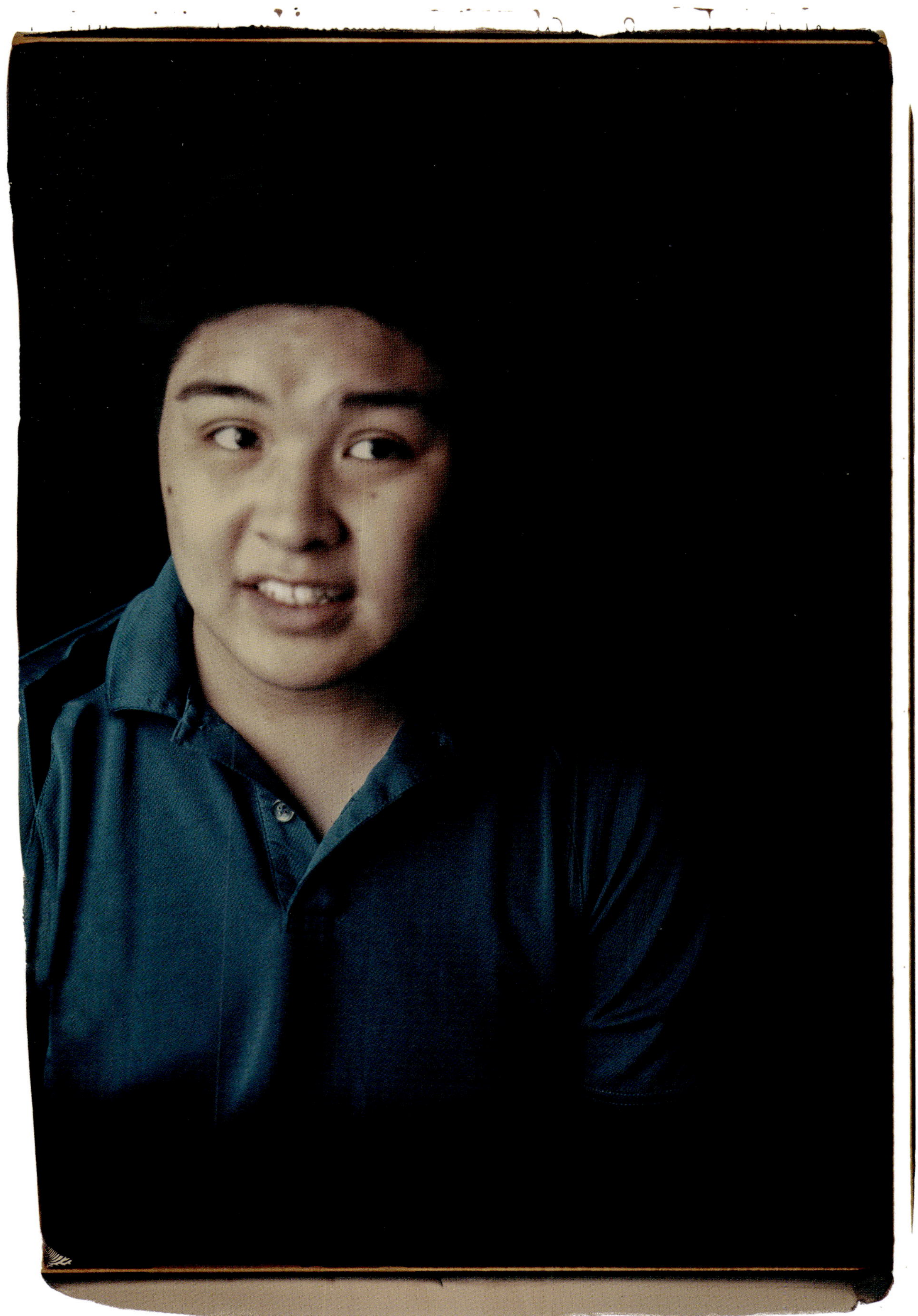

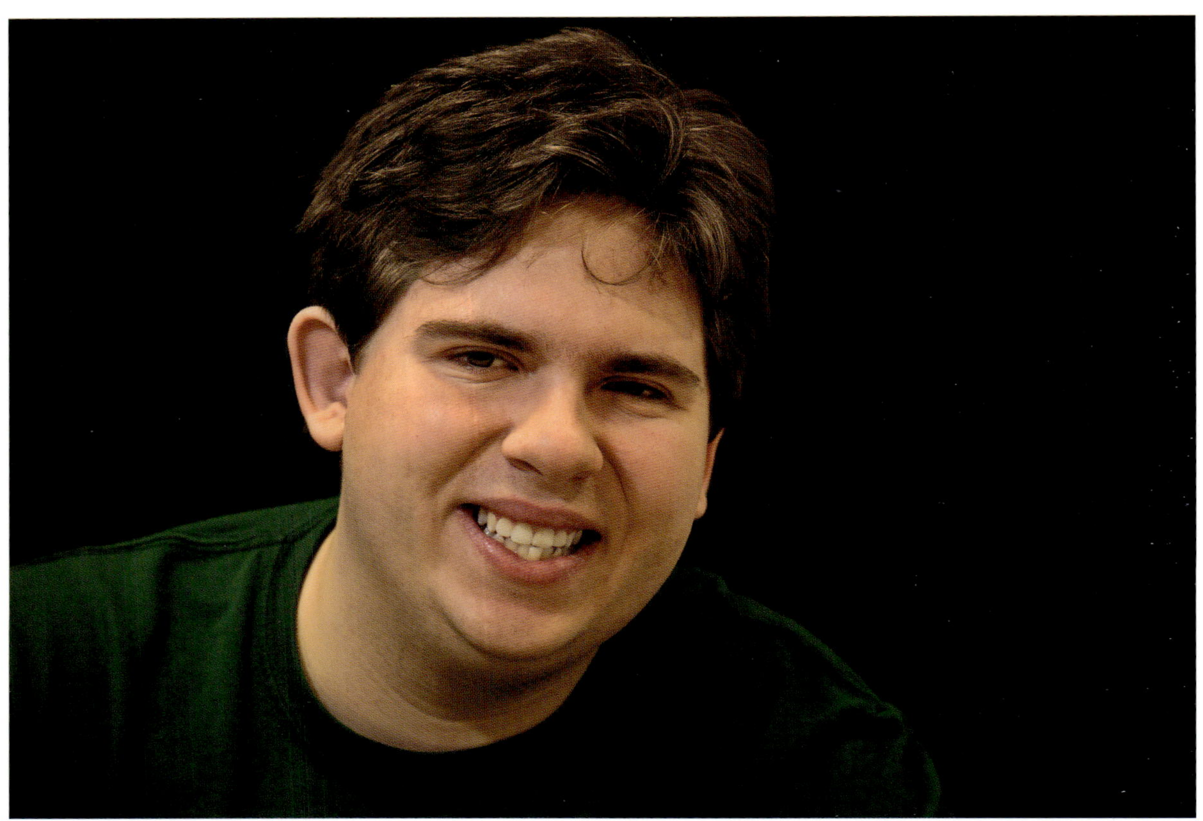

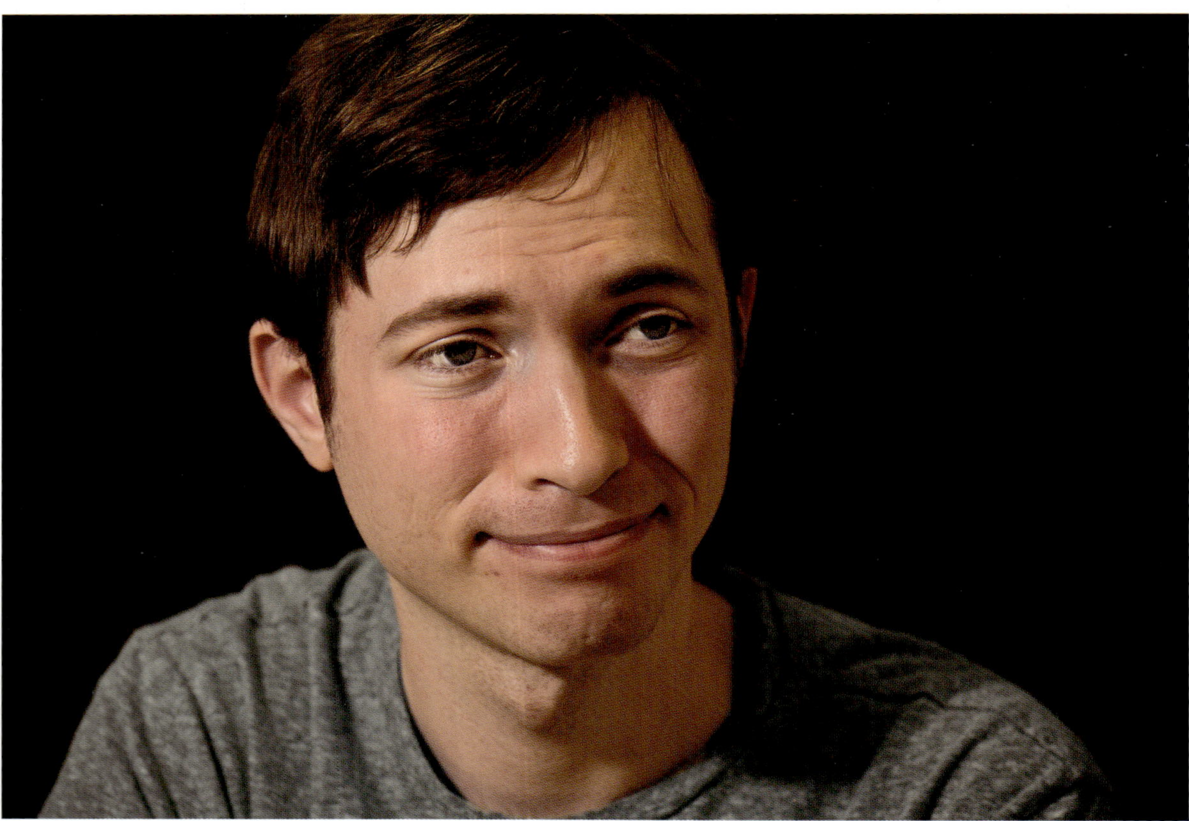

Top: Kenneth, *below:* Daniel

Kenneth & Daniel

twin brothers, at age 20

...they are as different as can be...

Our sons, Kenny and Danny, are fraternal twins, they are as different as can be — physically, emotionally, in their areas of interest, but they share a lot. They know a lot about each other naturally and they spend a lot of time together, which is a blessing.

Sometimes when we're together, Kenny unexpectedly turns to his brother. Kenny is about a half a foot shorter, and he reaches up and gives Danny a big kiss on his cheek, or a big hug. It's a beautiful thing.

~Hilary, Kenneth's and Daniel's mother

I just want people to accept them.

Danny has more language and he's starting to understand things better, so he sort of takes responsibility for Kenny. With Kenny, it takes a little time, but he gets it. He's coming along, he's doing good. He's certainly capable of the range of human emotion.

Kenny is happy when the family is together and we go places. He likes to try things. He loves museums, movies, vacations. He enjoys taking a walk or just being together. I think that's 'happy' for him.

I just want people to accept them and be patient with them. It's the same thing you want for anyone. You want people to provide them with the respect and the dignity they're due as human beings.

~Bob, Kenneth's and Daniel's father

A Few Closing Thoughts

We appreciate your taking the time to meet the young people of *Faces of Promise*. Their images and the words of their parents give us a glimpse of their dignity and beauty. They inspire us to do all that we can to contribute to greater awareness and understanding.

These young people deserve the full measure of acceptance in their schools and in their communities, as well as the opportunities that can enable them to make gains and experience a sense of accomplishment. Although strides have been made toward achieving these goals, it is still a work in progress. There are national and local autism organizations, schools, parent groups, places of worship, youth programs and many other organizations, large and small, who would welcome your participation and ideas.

Margaret Mead said, "Never doubt that a small group of thoughtful, committed citizens can change the world, indeed, it is the only thing that ever has."[1] This expression reminds me of the remarkable momentum that has been created by parents and other family members who have advocated for their children, and in so doing have touched the lives of many more children.

In some instances they have even established organizations that have developed strong voices. Their unstoppable commitment and that of other concerned citizens have greatly contributed to positive change.

With collective resolve, advocacy organizations and parent advocates, the scientific and university communities, public policy makers and legislators, nonprofit organizations, foundations, educators, clinicians and health care professionals have helped to move the autism agenda forward in support of individuals on the spectrum and their families. Efforts are ongoing to increase funding for basic and applied research; the development, expansion and access to evidence-based, scientifically validated programs and services; as well as the funding of these services for all. The ongoing call for action-oriented, autism public policy on local, state and national levels continues to be an important priority.

To date, all of these efforts have had, and continue to have, a significant impact, yet, there is much to be done. Each of us can take part in helping children, adolescents, young adults and adults on the spectrum to more fully realize their potential.

1 Nancy C. Lutkehaus, *Margaret Mead: The Making of an American Icon* (Princeton, NJ: Princeton University Press, 2008).

With Our Special Thanks

Our special thanks goes to all of the families who participated in *Faces of Promise*. Thank you so much for giving us the privilege to include your child and your poignant comments in our book that illuminates the dignity, beauty and promise of these children. And, a special thanks to the young people who shared their first-hand experiences with us.

Our appreciation to all those at *The Help Group* and *The Bay School* who participated in this project, and above all for their dedication and commitment to the children and their families.

We are most grateful to Pamela Clark, Director of *The Help Group's Autism Schools*, and Dr. Mary Bauman, *The Help Group* Clinical Director, for their invaluable input.

Our thanks to autism school administrators Andi Ambartsumyan, Dr. Ellis Crasnow, Sue Anne Kaples, Debbie Lazer, Dr. Sara McCracken, and Elena Ramirez for their ongoing involvement in this project, and to the teachers and teacher aides for lending a hand.

We'd like to acknowledge Dr. Andrea Gold, Executive Director of *The Bay School* in Santa Cruz, for her support of this project, and to Feda Almaliti, parent of a student at *The Bay School* and autism advocate, for her key role in the organization and participation of *The Bay School*.

The Help Group

Founded in 1975, *The Help Group* is one of the largest, most innovative and comprehensive nonprofits of its kind in the United States serving children, adolescents and young adults with special needs related to autism spectrum disorder (ASD), learning disabilities, attention deficit hyperactivity disorder (ADHD), developmental delays, abuse and emotional challenges. With a highly trained, interdisciplinary faculty and committed staff, its state-of-the-art schools and programs are located on five major campuses throughout The Greater Los Angeles Area.

The Help Group reaches more than 6,000 children and their families each year through extensive educational, mental health and therapy services, child abuse and residential programs. Its ten specialized day schools offer pre-K through high school programs, each based on the most current best practice models.

Recognized as a leader in the field of autism, *The Help Group's* six autism day schools serve more than 1,100 students ages 3–22 on a daily basis. The schools provide diagnostic prescriptive teaching; evidence-based, highly individualized curricula and intervention strategies; a high staff-to-student ratio; counseling; and speech, language and occupational therapy.

In addition, *The Help Group* offers a broad continuum of autism programs and services, including: assessment; early identification and intervention; therapeutic services; after-school enrichment; social skills clubs for teens and young adults; a therapeutic residential boarding school for adolescents; day and travel camps; pre-vocational and vocational training; life skills coaching; parent support groups; and a transitional residential program for young adults on a college campus.

The Help Group is widely regarded for its high standards of excellence and unique scope and breadth of services. Through its public awareness and outreach programs, university partnerships, applied research, graduate and postgraduate professional training, conferences and seminars, parent education programs, publications, and public policy efforts, *The Help Group* touches the lives of children with special needs and their families throughout the United States and in other parts of the world.

thehelpgroup.org

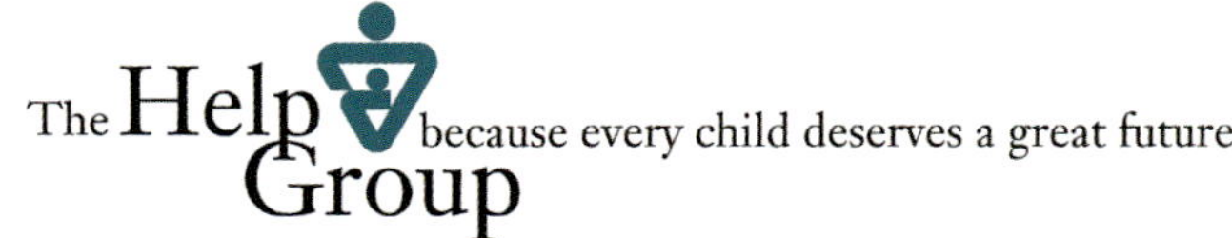

All of the students from The Help Group at the time of this publication had been attending or had graduated from one of the following Help Group schools.

Bridgeport School educates students ages 5 to 18 with mild to moderate cognitive delays and challenges with social communication and/or language development.

Bridgeport Vocational Education Center is designed for young adults ages 18 to 22 where they can develop the skills necessary for a successful transition to adulthood.

STEM³ Academy is the first school of its kind in the country to provide an innovative, rigorous STEM curriculum for students with social and learning differences, including autism.

Sunrise School serves students ages 5 to 22, with moderate to severe global delays associated with autism and other developmental disabilities.

Village Glen School is a college preparatory program serving students K–12 with challenges in the areas of socialization, pragmatic language development and peer relations.

Young Learners Preschool is an interdisciplinary early intervention day school program for children 2.9 through 5 years of age.

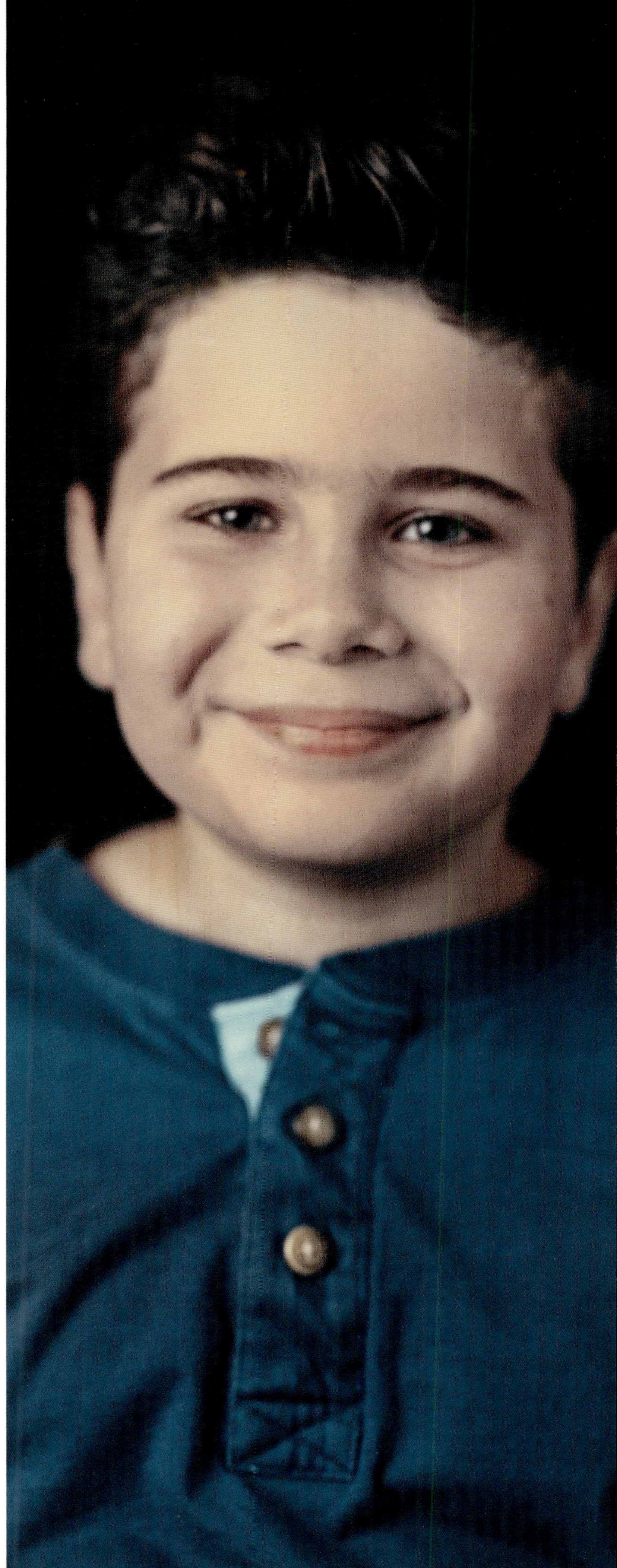

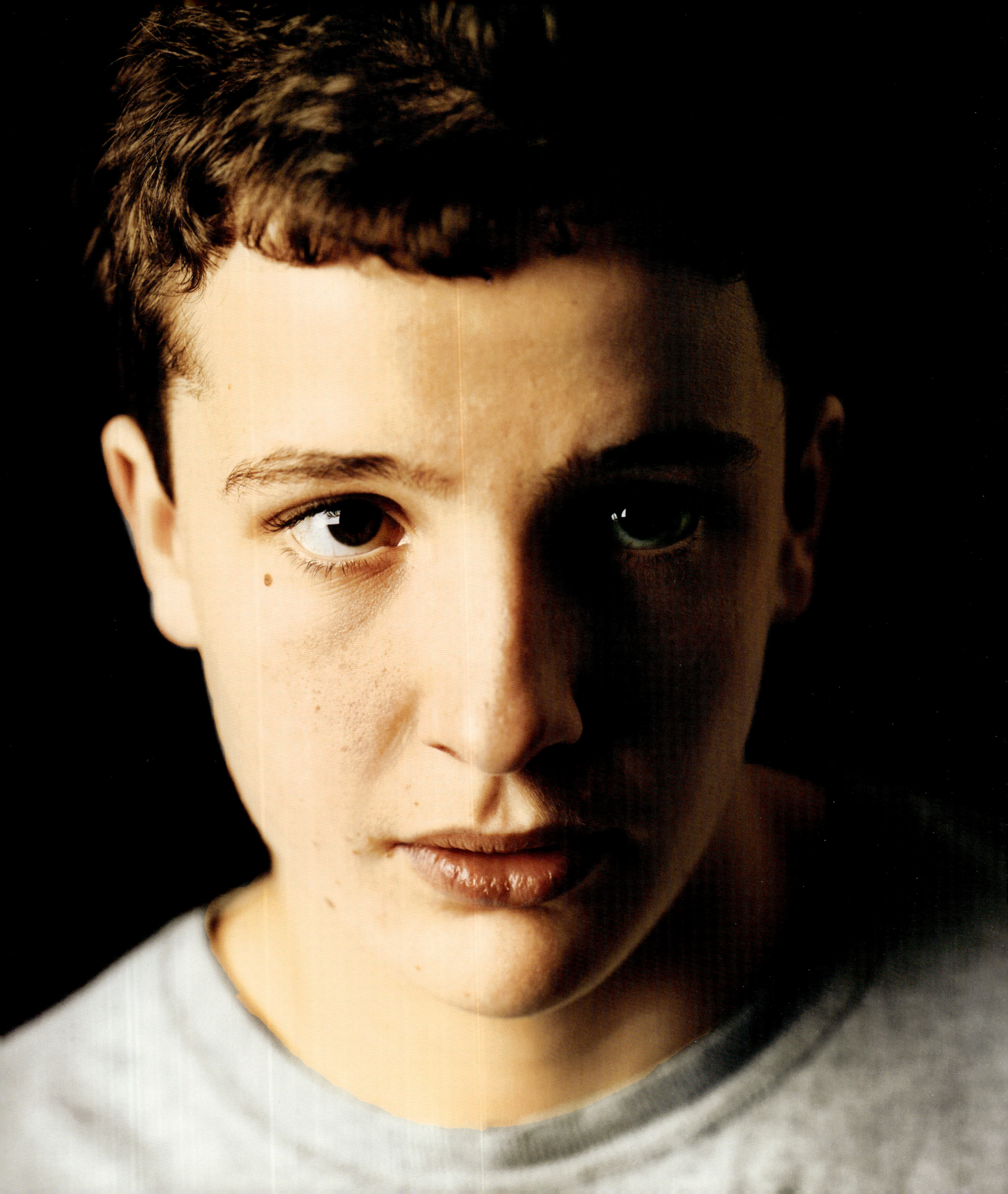

The Bay School

Founded in 1999, *The Bay School* is a nonprofit, nonpublic school located in Santa Cruz, California.

The Bay School provides students with autism and/or developmental disabilities ages 5 to 21 comprehensive, extended-year educational and clinical services regardless of their race, national or ethnic origin, age, gender, or religion. The educational and treatment approach used at *The Bay School* is based on the principles of applied behavior analysis, a methodology that applies principles of behavior to learning. Our mission is to provide scientifically-based educational and clinical services to produce measurable and lasting improvements in the lives of the students and families we serve.

The Bay School is part of the *May Institute*, a national organization of award-winning programs for children and adults with autism and other special needs.

The Bay School Offers

- An educational program that utilizes systematic instruction based on the principles of Applied Behavior Analysis
- Highly trained professionals seeking to improve the quality of life of the students in their care
- 1:1 staff-to-student ratio
- Curriculum that addresses the individual needs of each student
- Opportunities for research in areas of education and intervention for students with autism and/or developmental disabilities
- 12-month, full-day program

Student Education

Teaching programs are developed based on each student's educational and behavioral needs. Individualized educational plans are designed for each student with annual objectives and measurable outcomes.

Objectives emphasize the development of language skills, academic skills, social skills, leisure skills, and self-help and safety skills. Students' progress is closely monitored by detailed data collection.

We work closely with families and encourage them to observe their child in programming, attend parent meetings, and implement teaching procedures in the home.

Journey into Adulthood

Our focus is on helping our students successfully transition out of the classroom and into the community.

Our supported employment program offers our adolescents and young adults opportunities to engage in valuable volunteer or paid work experiences in integrated community work settings.

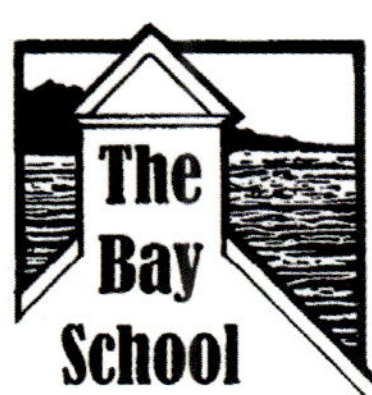

thebayschool.org

About Autism

For those of you who may be unfamiliar with autism, we'd like to share these basic facts with you.

Autism Spectrum Disorder (ASD), commonly referred to as autism, is a group of brain-based developmental disorders. Autism is a broad spectrum ranging from mild to severe. It is characterized by varying degrees of impaired social communication and interaction, and restricted, repetitive behaviors, interests or activities. These core symptoms can manifest themselves in behavioral challenges requiring different levels of support and intervention. No two individuals on the autism spectrum are the same. It is important to note that in addition to the core symptoms and other related challenges, children possess strengths and abilities.

Autism is estimated to affect 1 in every 68 children in the United States. It occurs in boys four to five times more frequently than in girls and impacts children from all ethnic, cultural and socioeconomic backgrounds. The estimated prevalence of autism has increased significantly since the 1990s. This increase has been influenced by greater awareness, improved expertise in diagnosis and an expanded definition. However, a component of true increase cannot be ruled out.

Autism may be accompanied by intellectual disability and language impairments. Some children are nonverbal or minimally verbal, but can learn to communicate through assistive technology.

In addition to the core symptoms of autism, individuals on the spectrum may experience associated medical conditions and other related challenges that may vary in severity.

Some children on the spectrum possess average to above average intellectual abilities. Other strengths can include excelling in math, science, music and art.

The causes of autism are unclear. Research suggests that the causes are complex and may include genetic, biological and environmental risk factors.

For many children, symptoms of autism can often be detected at 18 months or earlier, and can be reliably diagnosed by 24 months. Overall, children are typically diagnosed from three to five years of age, and in some cases, even later. When parents first suspect that their child is developing differently, they should discuss their concerns with their pediatrician and ask for an autism screening or referral to a qualified autism professional.

Early identification and intensive intervention based on best practices can result in significant positive outcomes for many children.

School-age children can benefit from evidence-based educational and therapeutic programs and services tailored to meet their individual needs.

When adolescents "age out" of the education system at 18 or 22 years old, they can benefit from services and support to help them transition to young adulthood and foster their ability to lead positive, productive and rewarding lives.

Individuals with autism can make gains throughout their lifetime with access to programs and services designed to maximize their strengths and help address their challenges.

For more information about autism and resources available, please visit

thehelpgroup.org

autismspeaks.org

nimh.nih.gov

cdc.gov

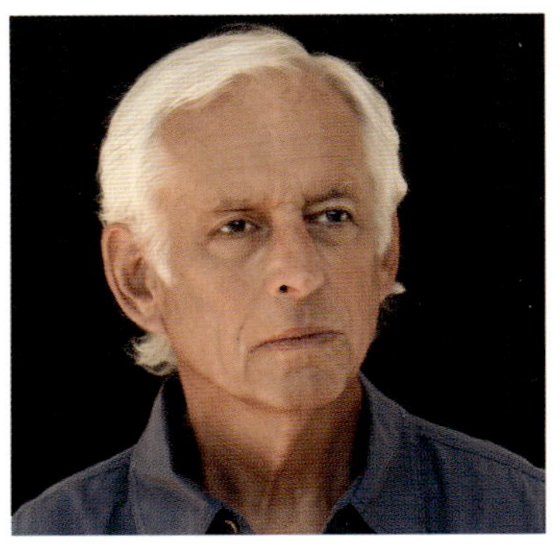

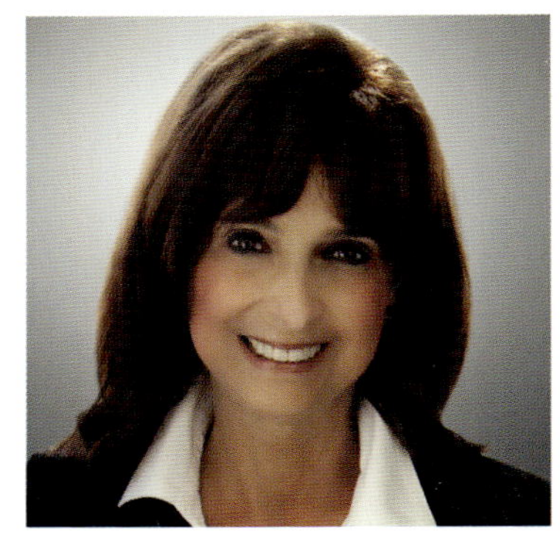

Richard Ehrlich, M.D.

Richard M. Ehrlich was born in New York City and resides in Los Angeles. Since 2001 his fine art photographs have been held in the permanent collections of nineteen museums, including the *Smithsonian National Museum of American History*, the *Los Angeles County Museum of Art*, the *UCLA Hammer Museum*, *The George Eastman House*, the *Denver Art Museum* and the *Santa Barbara Museum of Art*.

Ehrlich was the first to photograph the *Holocaust Archives* in Bad Arolsen, Germany. The project is part of the permanent collections of the *United States Holocaust Memorial Museum, Yad Vashem in Jerusalem, The Jewish Museum New York, The Jewish Museum Berlin,* and *Musée d'Art et d'Histoire du Judaïsme*, Paris, as well as others.

He has participated in over thirty–five gallery shows. His books include *The Forbidden Zone: Images from Namibia, Anatomia Digitale* (both from Nazraeli Press) and *Face The Music* (Steidl). *The Other Side of the Sky* and *Reverie* were also recently published. *Neogenesis* is to be published by Nazraeli Press in 2017. He was the photographer for *Decoding Mimbres Painting*, an exhibit and catalog to be showcased at LACMA January 2018. Steidl will publish *What's Past is Prologue: That Was Then, This is Now* in 2018.

Barbara Firestone, Ph.D.

Dr. Barbara Firestone is the President, CEO and Founder of *The Help Group*. Widely recognized for her vision and innovative spirit, she has dedicated her life's work to helping children with special needs realize their fullest potential. Under her leadership, *The Help Group* has become one of the nation's largest and most comprehensive nonprofits of its kind serving young people with autism and other special needs. With an impressive list of accomplishments and contributions to the field, Dr. Firestone has created brighter futures for countless young people.

Dr. Firestone is committed to promoting autism awareness, early identification and the development and expansion of education and treatment opportunities for children, adolescents and young adults. She has played a key role in California's autism public policy. She was appointed Vice Chair of the trailblazing *California Legislative Blue Ribbon Commission on Autism* and appointed to a leadership role in support of the *California Senate Select Committee on Autism & Related Disorders*.

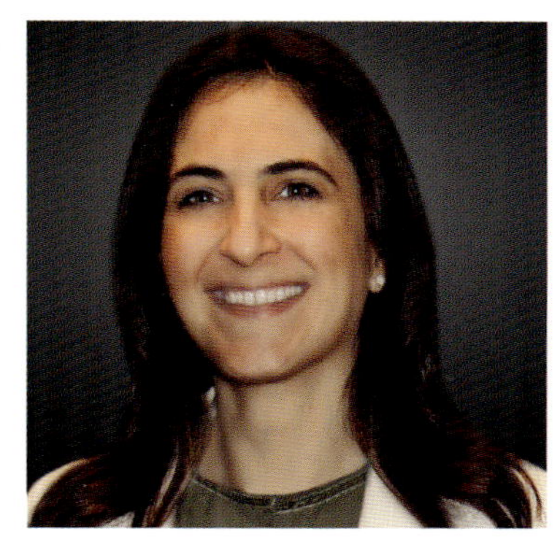

Lisa Manafian-Rozati

In the arena of professional training and research, Dr. Firestone collaborated with the *UCLA Semel Institute* to establish *The Help Group – UCLA Autism Research Alliance* and *The Help Group – UCLA Neuropsychology Program*, and with the *USC Chan Division* to launch *The Help Group – USC Occupational Science Initiative*.

To provide a lifeline of hope and support for families, Dr. Firestone wrote the highly acclaimed and award-winning book *Autism Heroes: Portraits of Families Meeting the Challenge*.

Lisa Manafian-Rozati, *Faces of Promise* coordinator, is *The Help Group's* Director of Special Projects and former Director of Communications. In her role, Lisa oversees a wide range of special projects and initiatives – the most recent include her development of an animal-assisted intervention program, her coordination of *The Help Group – USC Occupational Science Initiative*, and a collaboration with *Southern California Special Olympics* to establish a program at *The Help Group*.

In addition to special projects, Lisa lends her expertise to key communications, online and print publications, social media content and philanthropic, professional community events.

Lisa earned her Master of Science degree at *USC's Keck School of Medicine* and *Marshall School of Business in Global Medicine Management*. She is committed to promoting the health and well-being of children, particularly children with special needs.

Acknowledgments

My abiding and enduring indebtedness to
R. Mac Holbert, who has been the lynchpin and
mainstay of all my projects since the inception
of my photographic journey. His mastery of
composition, color, light, shadow and nuance is
well evidenced in the images you hold before
you. It is a distinct privilege to have his counsel
and long-term friendship.

Tracy Storer began working with the 20"x24"
Polaroid Cameras as a student in Boston in the
early 1980s, eventually becoming Director of
the Boston *20x24 Studio*, and later, opening
20x24 West. As one of only a handful of
20"x24" operators worldwide, he has provided
expertise to many luminaries and legends of
photography. His expertise has been invaluable.

I am indebted to Tyson Lee Smyer, our
indefatigable lighting specialist, who
transformed dark into light and was responsible
for the ability to capture the proper contrast
and luminosity of all these portraits.

Kudos to Lilla Hangay for her critical eye,
artistic sensibility and design expertise. Her
insights have been indispensable in shepherding
this project to its realization.

Ming Tshing, as always, provided superb technical
and special assistance.

Michael Friedman provided wise counsel
regarding all aspects of book publishing and
distribution for which we are extremely grateful.

Our special thanks to Max Herren for his superb
copy editing, and Karen Matsu Greenberg for
her outstanding production management of
this project.

Judie Garnett provided indispensable
managerial support.

Richard Ehrlich, M.D.

As always, I am most grateful to my husband, David, for his enduring support of my life's work that has meant so much to me throughout the years. He possesses a remarkable sensitivity for children with special needs and has given so much of himself on their behalf.

David and I are very proud of our family — Sarah and Jeremy Milken, Samantha and Jonathan Firestone, Shari Firestone and our grandchildren, Jake, Marin, Charlotte and Hudson — who all share in the core value of helping others.

With a sense of great appreciation, I'd like to acknowledge *The Help Group's* Board of Directors for its heartfelt and longstanding commitment to furthering *The Help Group's* endeavors that have created brighter futures for so many children.

The Help Group's Chief Operating Officer, Dr. Susan Berman has been integral to our efforts for the past 34 years. Her innovative leadership in the development of our autism programs provides help, hope and opportunity to young people on the spectrum.

For nearly 25 years, *The Help Group's* Senior Vice President Tom Komp has dedicated his invaluable expertise to *The Help Group* in many arenas. And, he has been a beacon of light and wisdom for countless families, offering his encouragement and guidance.

The Help Group has a terrific executive team, administration, faculty, staff and volunteers who help us to achieve our mission on behalf of the children and their families.

I'd like to acknowledge the following individuals for their contributions to *Faces of Promise*: Lisa Manafian-Rozati, *The Help Group's* Director of Special Projects and coordinator of *Faces of Promise*, for her expertise and dedication that has contributed greatly to bringing *Faces of Promise* to fruition.

Bradley Shahine, Director of Public Affairs, and Gerry Rosenblatt, long-time friend to *The Help Group*, have made meaningful contributions and have devoted many hours to this project.

My thanks to Camilo Vila, Kert Vandermeulen and Aldo Jimenez for their enthusiastic involvement as part of the *Faces of Promise* team.

Barbara Firestone, Ph.D.

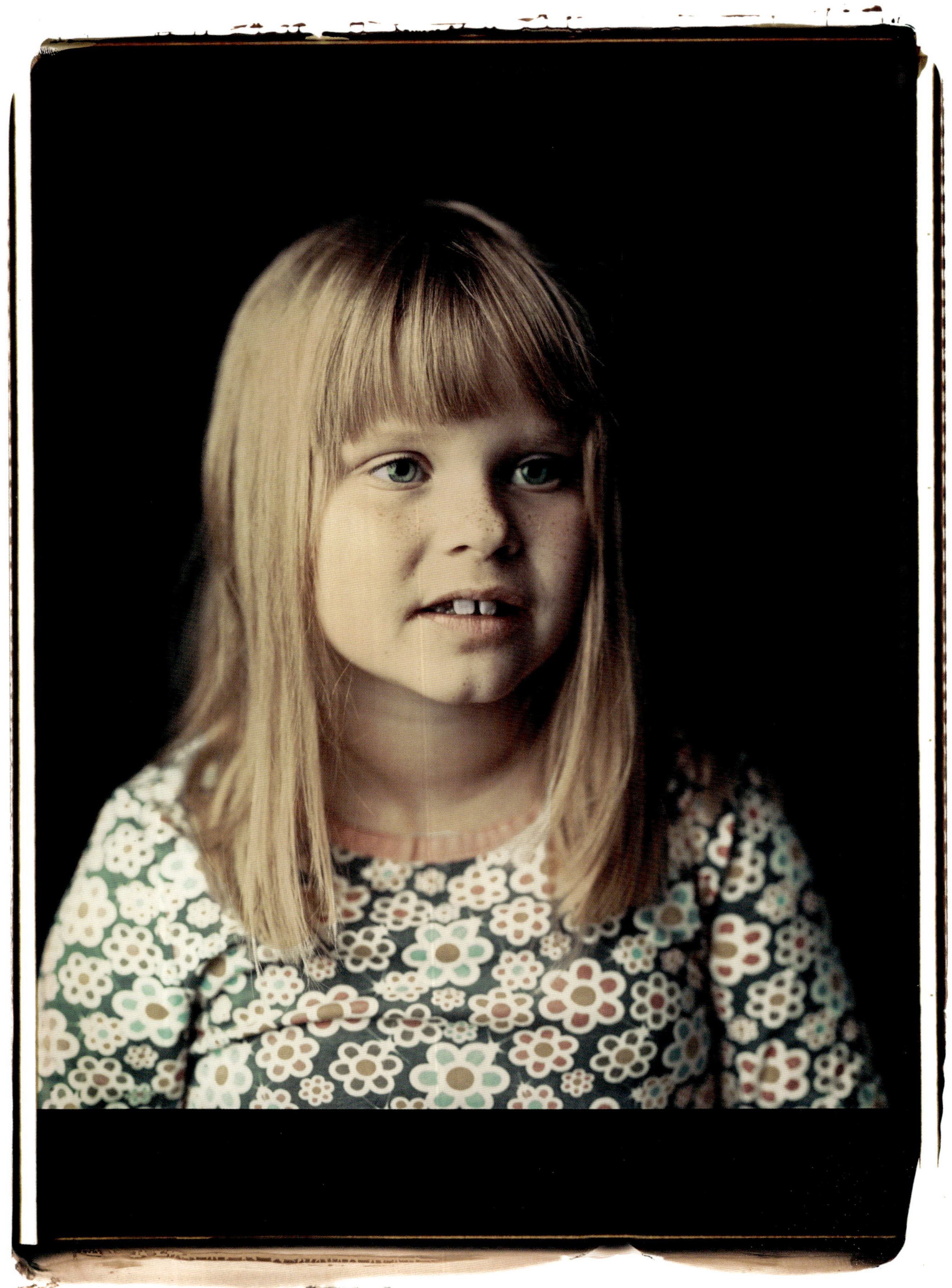

20"x24" Polaroid Camera

The 20"x24" Polaroid Camera, originally created in 1976, was the brainchild of the genius Edwin Land, the founder of Polaroid. Measuring over 6 feet tall and weighing 235 pounds, the camera typically operates in a studio but is occasionally transported to remote venues by truck.

It has been employed by many famous artists, such as Ansel Adams, Chuck Close, Andy Warhol, Robert Mapplethorpe, Mary Ellen Mark, William Wegman, Lucas Samaras and others.

It stands apart from other photographic media, not only by its sheer size and immediacy of printing, but by its arresting, ethereal high definition image capture. A close-up of a face can be much larger than life-size affording a surreal aura with striking color and clarity.

Worldwide there are currently only 3 cameras in use and unfortunately, at the end of 2017, the 20"x24" Polaroid Camera will become extinct, as the original Polacolor film will no longer be available, nor possible to replicate.

Richard Ehrlich, M.D.

Faces of Promise – Looking Beyond Autism
Richard Ehrlich / Barbara Firestone

Copyright © 2017 Richard Ehrlich / Barbara Firestone

First edition published by Graphic Arts Books
1700 Fourth Street, Berkeley, CA 94710
graphicartsbooks.com

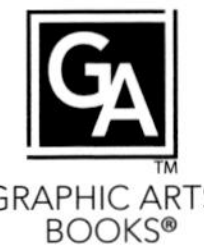

GRAPHIC ARTS
BOOKS®

Photography © Richard Ehrlich, M.D.
Text © Barbara Firestone / Richard Ehrlich
Epigraph: David M. Firestone

Faces of Promise was made possible in part through the
generosity of *The Richard Ehrlich Family Foundation* and
The From The Heart Charitable Trust.

Library of Congress Cataloging-in-Publication Data
available upon request.

ISBN: 978-1-513-26088-4

Printed in Singapore by KHL Printing Co Pte Ltd